D0000626

the
Fibromyalgia
Nutrition
guide

Mary Moeller, L.P.N.
and
Dr. Joe M. Elrod

WOODLAND PUBLISHING
Pleasant Grove, Utah

The information in this book is for educational purposes only and is not recommended as a means of diagnosing or treating an illness. All matters concerning physical and
mental health should be supervised by a health practitioner knowledgeable in treating
that particular condition. Neither the publisher nor author directly or indirectly dis-
pense medical advice, nor do they prescribe any remedies or assume any responsibility
for those who choose to treat themselves.

Contents

Foreword • 4

SECTION 1
Introduction • 5

SECTION 2
The Critical Nature of Food • 12
Balance and Variety: The Keys in Nutrition • 13
The Basic Foods • 16
The Miracle Nutrients • 20
Achieving and Maintaining a Healthy Weight • 30
Problems with Additives, Metals, and other Toxins • 3

SECTION 3
Flours and Grains • 43
Sweeteners • 52
Herbs • 56
Beginning Changes in Eating Habits • 64

SECTION 4
Recipes for Health • 69
Breads • 70
Desserts • 84
Fruit Sauces and Toppings • 103
Drinks • 105
Main Dishes and Soups • 111
Salads • 134
Dressings • 142
Vegetables • 145

Bibliography • 152
Resource List • 157
Other Resource Materials • 166

FOREWORD

There is no better way to learn about a health challenge than to know someone who has experienced it, or to be involved with someone who has learned to treat it. Mary Moeller first developed the symptoms of fibromyalgia when she was only 10 years old. But it wasn't until her daughter Kelly began having the same problems that she became motivated to help them both.

Mary and Kelly are now well. Nutritional intervention was a major part of their healing process. Now, after five years of feeling well, Mary has decided to share her story to and nutritional insights so that you, too, can begin the road to recovery from this debilitating syndrome.

The perception that fibromyalgia is "something you just have to live with" has been forever laid to rest by Dr. Joe Elrod and his research into fibromyalgia. In appearances all over the United States and internationally, Dr. Elrod has given hope to tens of thousands of patients who had previously felt that their diagnosis of fibromyalgia was little less than a sentence of chronic pain and restricted lifestyle with no hope of commutation.

After meeting in 1997, Mary Moeller and Joe Elrod became friends and collaborators, leading to this book long-awaited by the untold number of people who have repeatedly called, written, and essentially told them to "put it in writing."

As a physician, I owe a debt of gratitude to these two. They've enlightened me and inspired me to undertake their common task—to educate the 18,000,000 people who suffer from fibromyalgia in the U.S. and Canada. Just as the downward spiral to poor health once seemed unavoidable, now the climb back up that spiral to your former vital self will become the inevitable.

Rob Robertson, Jr., M.D.

Introduction

The current interest and attention given to natural healing, foods and herbs, is absolutely remarkable. Thirty years ago the idea of food and herbal therapy as a means of treating or preventing disease would not have been readily accepted. Credible professionals would have been very hesitant to recommend natural therapies.

The American people have brought about drastic change in the past twenty years by seeking all possible health-care options. Variables within our modern day society such as highly refined foods, air and water pollution, stress, and dependence on prescription drugs, have encouraged the investigation of natural approaches and remedies. We have become more and more aware that medical science alone does not necessarily hold all the answers to health and vitality.

MARY'S STORY: FIRST-HAND EXPERIENCE

Growing up on a farm in Northwestern Iowa was a wonderful experience. As a child, my hopes and dreams were to grow up on the farm, get married, and live my life as a farmer's wife. Each year I would raise a large garden, sheep and chickens. As a young child, I could have never known or understood what life actually had in store for me. It was good I had no understanding as to the pain and distress that lay ahead or how weak my little body would become. If I could have seen the future, I may have been tempted to give up.

As a two-year old, I remember spending many days at the doctor's office and in the hospital. It was during that year in my life I began gaining an unusual amount of weight, which brought a diagnosis of nephritis. After a bout in the hospital, my mother would drive me a mile and a half to a tiny town, which consisted of a tiny grocery store, grain store, and a gas station, to weigh me on the produce scale. I remember feeling very special sitting in that scale, although I didn't realize that each time I was set in that scale, my mother would fear the worst, which would be an extra pound of weight gain from the previous reading taken a short twelve hours before.

The doctors didn't offer much hope to my parents that I would make it through the disease, and on a number of occasions while I was in the hospital, they would call my parents in, expecting my little body wouldn't make it until the next day. Then came what would be the magic cure--penicillin. That "new" antibiotic would turn out to be my life savior, while at the same time, my curse. I continued taking penicillin until I was ten years old.

I continued to improve and become stronger. By the time I entered Junior High, I had become healthy and strong. I began playing sports and joined the school band. As with many children at that age, there was much stress, but overall, I learned to love life and everything it represented. It was also during that time that I began having sleeping problems. I had trouble getting to sleep and when I did get to a deep enough sleep, I would have horrific nightmares. It was diagnosed as "hormonal." Fibromyalgia was not in anyone's vocabulary in those days.

I was plagued with a feeling of tiredness, but I adjusted my body. When I entered high school, I began having trouble with my grades. When test day would arrive, I knew the chapters like the back of my hand, but I could not recall the information at test time. I did fairly well in sports and music, but I always had a sense of embarrassment when it came to the weekend. I wasn't allowed to participate in the sports or musical activity due to my failure of tests during the week. Due to my grade fluctuations, the doctor diagnosed me as depressed and suggested that I be taken out of any extracurricular activities until I got on top of things. I also developed stomach problems that were thought to be the beginning of ulcers.

When I graduated from high school, I hoped to become a cosmetologist. Due to a diagnosis of rheumatoid arthritis and irritable bowel syndrome, it was suggested that I choose another field. I chose the nursing field and proceeded to a junior college. I was still plagued with the memory problems. I learned in my freshman year that if the instructors wrote the information on the chalkboard, I could recall the information at test time. My grades were good enough to put me on the honor roll.

By the time I was 22, I felt as though my body was dying. I knew if I didn't do something soon, it would all end. I began riding my bicycle everyday. I would ride ten to forty miles a day. I thought this would make my body stronger. After four short months, my body did give out, and I was diagnosed with mononucleosis. It took about six months for my body to recover from that illness, after which I was diagnosed with that dreaded disease a second time, but this time it was back with a vengeance. Within a week of the second diagnosis, I was in the hospital. It was also determined that I had hepatitis. I was confined to my home for six weeks, any exercise activity was out of the question. I was having constant joint pain accompanying my illness.

My doctors, my family, and my friends were convinced that I was becoming a hypochondriac. I learned to keep aches and pains to myself. I became a "quiet sufferer."

In 1977, I met Karl Moeller and we married a few months later. In the first year of our marriage, I was diagnosed with endometriosis, and after two miscarriages, I carried our son to full term. Even though I felt better during the pregnancy than I had in years, the symptoms of fibromyalgia returned and were more severe. Pelvic pain, back pain, memory problems, sleeping difficulty, overall weakness, breast pain, and extreme fatigue made each day more and more difficult.

Due to the economy at that time, we moved seven times during the next five years. At the age of 29, I under went a hysterectomy and an appendectomy to alleviate the endometriosis. Three months after that surgery, I under went another surgery to remove a mass from my abdomen. In the year to follow, I had two more surgeries. One to remove non-malignant tumors from my breasts and the other to remove adhesions from my abdomen. I was suffering from severe back pain, constant upset stomach, bouts of diarrhea and constipation, bladder spasms, and heart palpitations. Muscle spasms and twitches consumed me every hour of every day. Sleep was nonexistent. Meals would take hours to prepare. I recall having to lay down on the kitchen floor to build up enough energy to finish preparing a simple meal.

In 1986, our baby girl from Korea arrived. Although a bit malnourished and tired, she was absolutely beautiful. Our family was now complete.

The pain was still prevalent, but had become accompanied by depression and horrific nightmares. It was at this time I was finally given a diagnosis for all of symptoms I had been plagued with. The diagnosis was fibrositis. It was suggested that the practice of yoga exercises may help keep my muscles strong and meditation would help with the pain. They both turned out to be very helpful.

We moved two more times in the next four years.The symptoms had become quite severe. My only relief came in exercise. Doctors had suggested to me that I could take up to 24 ibuprofen a day safely. Other than thinning my blood, it really did not accommodate the pain. Eating had become a double edge sword. My stomach felt better when I was hungry, but would soon become severely upset after I ate. I was now dealing with symptoms closely similar to those of someone that suffers from multiple sclerosis. Thankfully, I had a friend with MS to help me understand and who could sympathize with my condition.

We made our final move in 1990. That move would prove to be yet another step in a plan by a higher force than mine. The occupant of the home before us had planted mint beside the house. Only in my attempt to get rid of it did I discover the benefits for stomach problems like I had. I spent the next two years researching, studying, and planting my own herbs and using them for every symptom that I had.

In 1992, our daughter was diagnosed with fibromyalgia. Her symptoms were so severe, we were forced to remove her from public school. On two occasions they found her wandering aimlessly outside of the school building; her memory had become so terrible she didn't know where she was to go.

I knew I had to do something for her. So, I called my brother-in-law, Dr. Randy Dierenfield, who is an acupuncturist, a chiropractor, and a nutritionist. He felt those of us suffering with fibromyalgia have experienced some form of trauma, which causes the immune system to break down. Our goal was to create a lifestyle that would provide the body with everything necessary to rebuild the immune system. With his help, I began to change not only my lifestyle, but my daughter's as well. She was much better within six months, although it took me almost a year to become free of symptoms. At that time, we treated this as an immune system breakdown, although there was no substantial scientific evidence to our theory. Then, in the fall of 1997, I met Dr. Joe Elrod. Dr. Elrod had conducted extensive research in the field of fibromyalgia. In his work, he had found and proven our theory of an immune problem causing the symptoms of fibromyalgia. Finally, we had a proven answer as to why the changes Kelly and I made had worked.

Today, I enjoy a pain-free, healthy life. There are many people who comment on the way my family and I eat, but I tell them we eat just eat as nature intended. It's not a "chore" to live a more healthy lifestyle, but a way of life. God has taken me on a journey, one of great learning. I know He has been with me every step of the way, and that is why I am able to help and encourage everyone that is experiencing the same symptoms and "Hell" as I did. Many people will say to me that they could never give up chocolates, coffee, sugar, or soft drinks. They say it is the only enjoyment they receive in their life. I tell them that I can help them make a few changes to get their life back! Imagine yourself doing all of the things you once found near and dear to your heart. You can do those things! It only takes a little rearranging in your mind. By choosing to focus on the positives, you can gain a healthy lifestyle again! Allow all of those negative feelings about "changing" to fly away in the wind. Our hope is that this book provides you with the necessary information to make wise dietary changes that will lead to a happier, healthier life!

The Critical Nature of Food

Since you purchased this book, you are probably one of the millions of Americans who are not happy with what has happened to your health and your body for the past ten to twenty years. If that be the case, then consider this book a guide back to health and a lifelong prescription for a higher quality of life.

Would you be completely amazed if you were told that the selection, preparation and consumption of food is the key to your healing, energy and vitality?

Used correctly, food becomes the exceptionally powerful elixir that mankind has searched centuries for. It can keep you mentally clear and focused throughout the day. It can increase your physical stamina, leaving you with extra energy at the end of the day. Food used properly can also assist with continuous body cleansing, aid with stress coping and slow the aging process.

Finally, one of the most positive side effects of using food properly is the loss of excess body fat without the use of drugs or fad diets, which are extremely dangerous and unhealthy.

Always listen to your body after eating. It will tell you in subtle ways if a food you have eaten isn't beneficial. Many times those feelings will come before you begin to eat. You may see a food on the table and in your mind may think you you really shouldn't eat that food. Those feelings may be indicators your senses are trying to give you to help you know which foods on that table would be beneficial in your healing process and which would not be. Learn to listen to that inner voice inside of you that is there to help you to make the choices that will help your body to heal.

In both of our activities, the most frequent request from people like you has been to provide recipes and meal plans for those principles and guidelines. This book is an answer to that request. Hopefully, this book will help you develop habits necessary for your body to remain healthy and symptom free.

Balance and Variety: The Keys in Nutrition

Your body needs a variety of nutrients in order to function at peak performance, including fats, carbohydrates, protein, fiber, vitamins, minerals, and phytochemicals. In fact, the body needs 90 nutrients daily, including 60 minerals, 16 vitamins, 12 essential amino acids, and 3 essential fatty acids. A key to remember here is when treating fibromyalgia or any other chronic condition it is essential to eat a variety of food amounts and combinations. If one continuously eats the same foods over and over, one may miss out on many of the important building blocks in a healthful regimen. (Elrod, 1997)

The lower quality of our foods today enhance the weakening of our immune systems and increase the potential for chronic conditions such as fibromyalgia. In the past, more plants were organically grown and soils were much richer in a wider range of essential minerals. In today's commercial agriculture, healthy plants are artificially created by the use of herbicides, fungicides, fertilizers, and pesticides. When chemicals are sprayed on plants, essential soil microbes are killed that help plants absorb minerals into their root systems. So then, it is most difficult to absorb adequate levels of the essential nutrients when they are simply not available in the soil. Therefore, we should seek out more foods that are grown organically and that possess more of the vitamins and minerals without all the added chemicals (Weintraub, 1997).

EATING TO COMBAT FIBROMYALGIA

The most healthful eating patterns are to eat four to five, even six times daily, enjoying snacks (healthful snacks) for energy and nutrition. Never skip breakfast. Most unhealthy and/or overweight people develop the habit of skipping breakfast. Always eat the traditional breakfast, lunch, and dinner meals with a couple or three healthy snacks in between. The following are a few suggestions for eating throughout the day:

- Eat every few hours to maintain energy, to avoid getting too hungry, and to keep metabolism at its maximum.
- Nutritious snacks should be stashed both at work and at

home (i.e., raw fruits and vegetables, vegetable and fruit juices, dried fruit, whole grain crackers, bagels, unsalted nuts, pretzels, and popcorn without butter.

• When concerned about late morning and late afternoon snacks that might ruin your appetite for the good meal, choose a piece of fruit, whole grain bread sticks or crackers, or nibble on raw vegetables. If you will work toward eliminating sugared cereals, soft drinks, candy, cookies, food additives and preservatives, you can quickly enhance the turn-around of the fibromyalgia symptoms, especially pain and the inability to sleep more soundly.

• Remember that everyone should eat a wide variety of foods, focusing on the 90 nutrients needed daily. Most people will benefit from eating more fresh fruits and vegetables, seeds, nuts, cereals and whole grains. These foods and others to be listed later provide the necessary increased fiber and fluid, the higher quality fats, the complex carbohydrates, the necessary proteins, and the vitamins and minerals necessary for optimal health and for combating fibromyalgia symptoms. The following guidelines will outline some healthful suggestions for a balanced nutritional program:

• Complex carbohydrates should make up approximately 50-55 percent of your calories. Carbohydrates are, no doubt, one of the most important foods as they provide most of the fuel for the moving body and the working, healing muscles. (And remember that the fibromyalgia condition is primarily located within the muscles and connective tissues.) Remember that energy is one of the primary problems with the fibromyalgia patient and that complex carbohydrates taken in on a daily basis will increase and maintain a high energy level.

• Fat should make up approximately 20-30 percent of your calories. Although fat has been tabbed as the culprit in heart disease and obesity, it is a necessary component in a healthful nutrition regimen. It is essential here to read your labels and get most of your fat from healthy sources such as polyunsaturates and monounsaturates such as canola, olive, safflower, peanut, and corn oils.

- Protein is also essential for balance, however, it should make up only 10-15 percent of your calories. Include protein from beans, legumes, nuts, other vegetables along with chicken, turkey, tuna, and fish. Utilize these sources of protein, rather than red meats which, in my opinion and as a result of research, is a detriment to the fibromyalgia victim.
- Avoid junk or fast foods and keep your diet very high in vegetable proteins. A very good suggestion would be to have a green salad and a portion of some type of beans everyday.
- By all means use purified water, ideally 8-10 eight-ounce glasses per day. A water purification system in the home is highly desirable to provide the pure water for cooking and drinking.
- It is essential to remove as many artificial food additives and chemicals as possible from your nutritional program.
- Avoid caffeine, sugar, and any unnecessary drugs not pre-scribed by your physician.
- Avoid refined and processed foods as much as possible, especially foods that are canned or boxed as they always have more additives. Fresh foods always have fewer addi-tives and sometimes will have none at all (Elrod, 1996).

The Basic Foods

In this section we will summarize the basic foods that form the foundation for your health and wellness.

For the past thirty years Americans have been led to believe that fat is the problem with our state of obesity and ill health. Ironically, the fact is that we are consuming less fat than ever before, yet systemic conditions such as obesity, diabetes, fibromyalgia and others are more prevalent than ever. Research scientists are pointing to the fact that this prevalence of obesity will serve to be the precursor to an unprecedented increase in chronic disease in our future.

Fat, carbohydrate, and protein constitute the three food groups. What the better sources of these groups are and an understanding of how they are to be balanced are the keys to restoring your health and staying healthy.

FATS

Fat is a most critical component of your nutritional program, therefore, the answer to being lean and healthy is definitely not to remove all fat from your diet. Fat performs as a control factor, slowing the rate at which carbohydrates enter the blood stream, thereby providing hormonal balance, specifically the decrease of the production of insulin. Fat is an important factor for reducing insulin and controlling weight.

There are basically three types of fat: saturated, which becomes solid at room temperature, monounsaturated and polyunsaturated, which remain liquid at room temperature. An example of saturated fat is butter, which is a much better choice over margarine. The best choices nutritionally are the monounsaturated and polyunsaturated fats such as olive oil and canola oil.

Fat plays some very critical roles such as slowing the rate of the absorption of carbohydrate into the bloodstream. Secondly, the proper balance of fat in the cells (all cells are composed of fat) allows membranes to perform at optimal efficiency. Finally, fat provides the essential fatty acids which are the building blocks of the most important hormones in the body called eicosanoids. This delicate balance of eicosanoids determines whether the body works efficiently and stays disease free. There are good and bad eicosanoids just as there is good and bad cholesterol. Another point in the critical importance of fat lies in the fact that the ratio of insulin and glucogon in your bloodstream determines whether your cells produce good or bad eicosanoids. Glucagon is a mobilization hormone that assists your body to use stored fats and carbohydrates for needed energy.

CARBOHYDRATES

Sources of carbohydrates are fruits, vegetables, and grains such as breads, pastas, and cereals. It is interesting to note that the body can manufacture carbohydrate, which is necessary for brain function, from protein and fat. This is not true for protein and fat, the human body cannot manufacture protein (the essential amino acids) or fat (the essential fatty acids), both must be obtained in the diet.

A complex carbohydrate is a group of simple sugars strung together by oxygen bonds. These carbohydrates can be absorbed only when the oxygen bonds are broken down to simple sugars in the stomach. This is very critical as it's the combination of the amount of carbohydrates you eat and how fast they are broken down to enter the bloodstream that determines how much insulin is produced.

Remember that insulin is a storage hormone as opposed to glucagon which is a mobilization hormone. One of the critical functions of insulin is to force new calories into the cells. The excess carbohydrates and protein converted to fat are driven by insulin into your fat cells for storage.

As you can readily see, the balance of fat, carbohydrate, and protein that you ingest on a daily basis is critically important, not only to a healthy weight but also to your general health and vitality.

PROTEIN

Protein is essential to life although you need less than either fat or carbohydrate. The key to our program is that you have adequate amounts of protein, not too little and not in excess. We lose protein daily through normal metabolism for energy. Therefore, the body cells, enzymes (the engines of life) in each cell, the immune system, and the levels of muscle mass all are dependent on adequate levels of new incoming protein on a daily basis.

Protein is derived primarily from animal sources. Unfortunately, protein levels in plants are generally very low requiring unrealistic and tremendous amounts of vegetables in order to get adequate protein. Much of the health problem in industrialized countries results from eating too little protein and by consuming more and more grains and pasta in an attempt to lower the amount of fat consumed.

The danger here is that inadequate protein leads to a weakened immune system that loses its ability to fight off foreign invaders and to combat infection. A lack of protein also causes a loss of muscle mass as the body will pull from existing muscle to meet the demand for amino acids to manufacture new essential enzymes and to boost the immune system. This creates a vicious cycle healthwise as reduced muscle mass lowers metabolism. As lean muscle mass decreases and fat content increases (due to a lower metabolism) the human health state deteriorates.

As stated earlier in the fat section, you want to keep the amount of saturated fat to a minimum. Therefore, the best sources of protein will be chicken, turkey, tuna, fish, cottage cheese, soybean-imitation meats, and tofu as opposed to sausage, beef and bacon.

Finally, a critical role of protein is that it stimulates the release of the hormone glucagon. Glucagon is the hormone that assists the body in utilizing essential fat and carbohydrates as energy sources.

Through the discussion above you can readily see why my program calls for the proper balance of fat, protein, and carbohydrate. We have referred to the better sources of the good fats, protein, and complex carbohydrates. A healthfully balanced nutrition program would be 10 to 15 % protein, 20 to 30% fat, and 50 to 55% complex carbohydrate, depending on body type, body chemistry, and metabolism.

The Miracle Nutrients

In this segment we will discuss some of the better sources of antioxidants, vitamins, minerals, enzymes, and other supplemental miracle nutrients. The more powerful antioxidant vitamins are beta carotene, vitamin C, vitamin E, and vitamin B6. Some of the trace minerals that serve as powerful antioxidants are selenium, zinc, manganese, magnesium, boron, and chromium. Some other powerful antioxidant and immune boosting nutrients are proanthocyanidins (from grape seeds), curcumin, and garlic. The foods and supplements that can provide the above miracle nutrients are very powerful weapons for fighting against and buffering free radicals and the damage they can deliver. The following are some excellent sources for the miracle nutrients in the preceding sections. (Elrod, 1997)

Beta Carotene: There are dozens of carotenoids of which beta carotene is one in the plant form of vitamin A. The better sources of carotenoids are yellow and orange fruits and vegetables such as carrots, cantaloupe, sweet potatoes, pumpkin, apricots, and melons such as mango, papaya, peaches and winter squash. The dark green leafy vegetables are another excellent source of beta carotene. Examples are collard greens, parsley, spinach, and broccoli.

Vitamin C: This is one of the more powerful antioxidants and the major sources are fresh fruits such as grapefruit, strawberries, bananas, cantaloupe, papaya, kiwi, mango, raspberries, pineapple, and tomatoes, as well as fresh vegetables such as cabbage, asparagus, broccoli, Brussels sprouts, collard greens, potatoes, and red peppers. Vitamin C is heat sensitive and easily destroyed by refining or over-processing. Therefore vegetables should be steamed or microwaved for a very short period of time.

Vitamin E: The better sources for this powerful antioxidant are vegetable oils, especially safflower, avocados, nuts, sunflower seeds, wheat germ, whole grain cereals and breads, asparagus, dried prunes, and broccoli.

Selenium: There is much evidence to substantiate that selenium boosts the immune system by protecting cells from the toxic effects of free radicals. Some of the better food sources of selenium are shrimp, sunflower seeds, wheat breads, tuna and salmon.

Zinc: This trace mineral assists in performing many of the vital body functions. For instance, it helps with the absorption of vitamins in the body and helps form skin, nails, and hair, as well as being an essential part of many enzymes involved in metabolism and digestion. Vitamin A must be present for zinc to be properly absorbed in the body. Some excellent sources of zinc are ginseng, chalk, and the herb licorice.

Manganese: A trace mineral essential for the proper functioning of the pituitary gland as well as healthy functioning of the body's other glands. It is essential in the treatment and healing of fibromyalgia in that it is an excellent aid in the utilization of glucose in the process of creating energy and it also helps in the normal functioning of the central nervous system.

Magnesium: This is a very essential part of the enzyme system and is seemingly most important in the rehabilitation from fibromyalgia. Almost 100 percent of the fibromyalgia victims with which I have worked have exhibited a magnesium deficiency. Another critical function of magnesium is in the absorption of potassium, calcium, phosphorus, the B complex vitamins, as well as vitamins C and E. Magnesium is also essential in ATP (energy) production.

Malic Acid: Another essential ingredient in the energy production process. Critical in lessening the toxic effects of aluminum. When combined with magnesium, malic acid is very effective as a cleansing and healing agent for fibromyalgia and other systemic conditions.

Chromium: This trace mineral is essential for the synthesis of fatty acids and the metabolism of glucose for energy. It is also well known for its ability to increase the efficiency of insulin.

Boron: This trace mineral possesses some antioxidant functions and is very important in maintaining muscular health in that it assists in inhibiting cells from releasing free radicals. Cauliflower and apples are sources of boron.

Proanthocyanidins: One of the potent sources of proanthocyanidins is grapeseed extract. Otherwise known as pycnogenol, proanthocyanidins are a very powerful antioxidant and are 50 times stronger than vitamin E. They are also very efficient in boosting the immune system and assisting in the treatment of fibromyalgia.

Glucosamine: The key substance that determines how many

proteoglycan (water holding) molecules are formed in cartilage. Glucosamine has been found to be very effective for improvement in arthritic conditions. Also, in a study conducted by the Vulvodynia Project, it was used to effectively reduce sensitivity and pain in soft tissue areas of fibromyalgia patients.

Calcium: Calcium is critically essential because it is the most abundant mineral in the body. Most of the calcium in the body is located in the bones and the teeth. It is necessary for the transmission of nerve signals and important for the smooth functioning of the heart muscles and muscular movements of the intestines. It is very important for good health, especially if one has a poor diet, suffers from malabsorption, or gets little sunshine. Calcium should be balanced with magnesium for proper nerve function and for a healthy body. Calcium, magnesium, and zinc all have a calming effect in the body and are very effective if taken before bedtime to help relax muscles and promote sleep. Vitamins A, C, D and phosphorus are also essential for the efficient functioning of calcium. Some of the symptoms of a calcium deficiency are tingling of the lips, fingers and feet, leg numbness, muscle cramps, and sensitivity to noise. (Note: Do not take antacids to make up for calcium deficiency.)

Potassium: Potassium is responsible for normal heart and muscle function, normal transmission of nerve impulses, and normal growth. It works with sodium to regulate the flow of nutrients in and out of the cells and also helps to stimulate the kidneys, keep the adrenals healthy, and is involved in the maintenance of heart rhythm. Potassium is vital in stimulating nerve impulses which cause muscle contraction. The symptoms of a potassium deficiency include muscle twitches, weakness and soreness, erratic and/or rapid heartbeats, fatigue, glucose intolerance, nervousness, high cholesterol, and insomnia.

B-Complex Vitamins: Fibromyalgia patients need more B vitamins since they are under a great deal of stress and B vitamins assist in the calming process and good mental health. They are also vital in the production of serotonin, a chemical in the body that influences calming behavior. When B vitamins are deficient due to inadequate nutrition or increased demand it can significantly contribute to the lack of an ability to handle stress. B-complex vitamins work together to calm the nervous system and support correct brain function as well as to improve concentration and memory. Much care should be taken when taking the B vitamins as too much vitamin B6 is capable of causing a folic acid deficiency.

Vitamin B1 (Thiamine): Vitamin B1 is necessary for digestion, blood cell metabolism, muscle metabolism, pain inhibition, and energy. B1 is a water soluble vitamin and needed in only small amounts on a daily basis. Some good sources of B1 are rice bran, wheat germ, oatmeal, whole wheat, sunflower seeds, brewer's yeast, and peanuts. Herbs that contain vitamin B1 are gotu kola, kelp, peppermint, slippery elm, and ginseng.

Vitamin B2 (Riboflavin): Vitamin B2 is necessary for antibody formation, red blood cell formation, cell respiration, fat and carbohydrate metabolism. B2 is also water soluble and must be replaced on a daily basis. It is also essential for proper enzyme formation, normal growth, and tissue formation. Some good sources of vitamin B2 are wild rice, liver, fish, white beans, sesame seeds, wheat germ, and red peppers. A few of the herbs containing B2 are gotu kola, kelp, peppermint, and ginseng.

Vitamin B3 (Niacinamide): Vitamin B3 assists the body in producing insulin, female and male hormones, and thyroxine. B3 is also needed for circulation, acid production, and histamine activation. Some good sources of vitamin B3 are white meat, avocados, whole wheat, prunes, liver, and fish. Symptoms of a B3 deficiency are hypoglycemia, memory loss, irritability, confusion, diarrhea, ringing in the ears, depression, and insomnia.

Vitamin B6 (Pyridoxine): Vitamin B6 is helpful in converting fats and proteins into energy and with the production of red blood cells. It is also essential for proper chemical balance in the body. B6 is especially helpful to the fibromyalgia sufferer who is experiencing excessive stress. Symptoms of a B6 deficiency include irritability, nervousness, depression, muscle weakness, pain, headaches, PMS, and stiff joints.

Vitamin B12 (Cobalamin): Vitamin B12 is essential for iron absorption; fat, protein, and carbohydrate metabolism; blood cell formulation; and long life of cells. A strict vegetarian will need to supplement with vitamin B12. Some symptoms of a B12 deficiency include headaches, memory loss, dizziness, paranoia, muscle weakness, fatigue, and depression.

Biotin: Biotin is especially needed if you are under excessive stress, experiencing malabsorption, or have a poor nutrition program. Biotin aids in protein, fat, and carbohydrate metabolism, fatty acid production, and cell growth. Some of the symptoms of a biotin deficiency are muscle pain, nausea, anemia, fatigue, high cholesterol, and depression.

Pantothenic Acid: Pantothenic acid is needed for the normal functioning of muscle tissue and protects membranes from infection. It is also essential for energy conversion, blood stimulation, and detoxification. Individuals under excessive stress and with poor diets need pantothenic acid to assist in normal body functioning. Symptoms of a deficiency include digestive problems, muscle pain, fatigue, depression, irritability, and insomnia. Pantothenic acid is vital for the fibromyalgia sufferer due to the above facts.

Para Aminobenzoic Acid (PABA): PABA assists in facilitating protein metabolism, promoting growth, and blood cell formation. Some of the symptoms of a PABA deficiency are depression, fatigue, irritability, nervousness, constipation, and, in the long run, arthritis.

Vitamin P (Bioflavonoids): Bioflavonoids work together with vitamin C to strengthen connective tissue and capillaries. Bioflavonoids are also essential to assist the body in utilizing most of the other nutrients. Good sources of bioflavonoids are spinach, cherries, rosehips, citrus fruits, apricots, blackberries, and grapes. Herbs that contain bioflavonoids are paprika and rosehips.

Melatonin: In the 1950s scientists discovered melatonin, a hormone which may be the partial answer to sleep problems. It may also may have the capability to affect other common distresses such as lack of immunity, aging, and cancer. Melatonin is produced by a small gland found in the center of the brain, the pineal gland. The pineal gland releases melatonin when the eye is not receiving light. Melatonin controls our sleep cycles and helps us to rest soundly. Another tremendous benefit of melatonin is that it contains vitamin E, one of the more powerful antioxidants and free radical fighters.

Valerian: Valerian is probably the herb most widely used for anxiety and nervous tension. It is used as a natural sedative to improve the quality of sleep and relieve insomnia and is also used to combat depression. Valerian contains essential oils and alkaloids which reportedly combine to produce the calming, sedative effect. Considered a nervine herb, it is used as a very safe non-narcotic herbal sedative and has been used for after-pains in childbirth, heart palpitations, muscle spasms, and arthritis. Valerian is rich in calcium, which accounts for its ability to strengthen the spine, nerves, and brain. It is also high in magnesium, which works with calcium for healthy bones and the nervous system. It is also very high in selenium and manganese to strengthen the immune system and contains zinc and vitamins A and C.

Pau d'Arco: Pau d'arco is reported to be a natural blood cleanser and builder. It also possesses antibiotic properties which aid in destroying viral infections in the body. It helps combat cancer and has been used to strengthen the body, increase energy, and strengthen the immune system.

Vanadium: There is not a great deal of information available on vanadium, yet much evidence points to the fact that this trace mineral probably assists in preventing heart disease. Vanadium is a cofactor to insulin and, along with chromium, is very efficient in breaking down fats and sugars helping to keep coronary arteries clear. This mineral is vital in the creation of energy.

Bovine Cartilage: A natural source used in the body to manufacture cartilage components necessary for joint and tissue repair.

Colostrum: The first milk provided by a mother for her newborn; colostrum provides proteins that "educate" or train the various immune cells to combat various diseases and chronic conditions.

5-Hydroxytryptophan (5-HTP): A valuable phytonutrient that has been shown to be effective against conditions like chronic fatigue syndrome and fibromyalgia. This includes reduction of pain, anxiety, and fatigue. 5-HTP has also been used for improving quality and quantity of sleep.

VITAMINS/MINERALS/NUTRIENTS MAXIMUM DAILY DOSAGE

The following is a table of the essential nutrients and recommended dosages for fibromyalgia and related systemic conditions:

ESSENTIAL NUTRIENT	RECOMMENDED DOSAGE
Beta Carotene	25,000 IUs
Vitamin C	1,000-3,000 mg
Vitamin E	400-800 IUs
Selenium	200 mcg
Zinc	30 mg
Magnesium	200 mg
Manganese	10 mg
Chromium	200 mcg
Pycnogenol	50 mg
Boron	3 mg
Malic Acid/Magnesium Oxide (taken in 4-6 doses)	400 mg
Glucosamine	1,000-1,500 mg
Vitamin B6 (pyrodoxide hydrochloride)	5 mg
Vitamin B12	200 mcg
Vanadium	20 mcg
Biotin	100 mcg
Niacin (niacinamide)	30 mg
Inositol	20 mg
Bovine cartilage	200 mg
Flaxseed oil (alpha linolenic acid)	800 mg
Evening primrose oil (gamma linolenic acid)	200 mg
Conjugated linoleic acid	225 mg
Colostrum	200 mg

As mentioned earlier, it is generally best to get vitamins, minerals, antioxidants, and the nutrients the body needs from fresh whole foods (ideally organic foods) rather than supplements. However, it is common knowledge that the proper amounts of vitamins, minerals, and nutrients are very difficult to acquire from foods because of depleted soils and the use of chemicals in the form of pesticides and insecticides. In order to get all of the necessary nutrients in today's world it is absolutely essential that supplements are taken, especially when treating chronic conditions such as fibromyalgia.

Is nutritional supplementation really necessary for healing and health? The answer is an unequivocal "yes." A well controlled study performed at the Shriner's Burn Trauma Center at the University of Cincinnati Medical School demonstrated conclusively that burn trauma victims of children's age faired far better when given extra nutritional supplementation over and above the normal "well-balanced diet" generally prescribed by practitioners. One hundred percent of the children receiving the extra supplementation lived, whereas tragically 44 percent of the children who were given the regular traditional medically and so-called balanced diet alone died. The scientists stated that, "To our knowledge this is the first controlled study to demonstrate what has been suspected and accepted for some time, that nutritional intervention improves survival."

MUSCLE/CONNECTIVE TISSUE AND BIOFLAVONOIDS

There are literally thousands of different types of bioflavonoids. They are found in virtually all plant foods and are essential for healthy capillary walls, the metabolism of vitamin C, and enhancing the utilization of other essential nutrients. The bioflavonoids aid fibromyalgia victims by:

• Enhancing the strength of collagen in connective tissue
• Strengthening muscle fiber
• Buffering free radical damage
• Enhancing the functioning ability of muscle fiber
• Enhancing the energy production process
• Enhancing the utilization of other nutrients in the body

Some excellent sources of bioflavonoids are fresh fruits and vegetables, seeds, nuts, legumes, whole grains, citrus fruits, onions, berries, green tea, and especially fruits that contain a pit (such as plums and cherries). There are also rosehip bioflavonoids as well as citrus bioflavonoids such as catechin, hesperidin, rutin, quercetin, milk thistle seed extract, ginkgo biloba extracts, pycnogenol (from grape seed extract), and rice bran extract (Carper, 1995).

Achieving and Maintaining a Healthy Weight

Being overweight is directly related to at least sixty-seven other diseases; specifically high blood pressure, heart disease, diabetes, secondary osteoarthritis, fibromyalgia, stress and depression. By employing a good weight maintenance program or by reducing your weight (if you are overweight) you can greatly improve the symptoms of fibromyalgia. Remember a healthy weight is one of the major components of your health and wellness program during the healing and recovery process.

Following highly restrictive diets or crash diets that are based on a limited number of foods are not healthy physiologically and basically do not work in the long run. On many of these diets you will almost always lose weight initially, and sometimes a great deal of weight in the first week or two, and feel that you are beginning a program on which you are highly successful. However, again, these programs are not healthy and do not work for the long term. Research studies show that people who go on the stringent or highly restrictive diets usually lose weight but then gain it over and over again. These people normally become fatter over the long haul and also have a higher mortality rate than those who remain at a constant weight on a very healthy weight maintenance program. This is why it is very important to make a lifestyle change where you are adhering to healthful lifestyle prescription on a daily basis. This can really make the difference for health and longevity. A key is to choose a very easy, flexible, sensible nutrition plan that does not call for special shopping or tedious calorie counting, such as the plan provided for you here.

The following are a few guidelines to assist you along the way on your sensible, flexible and healthful lifetime weight management program. The individuals who have lost weight successfully and kept it off have generally utilized the following guidelines:

- *Make a commitment to change.* Without a firm commitment, chances for change are not very likely. This must be your goal to improve your health, lose weight, and reduce the symptoms of your fibromyalgia. If this is the goal of your physician or a family member, but not your own, then it's not likely that you'll be successful.
- *Plan ahead and be organized.* Do not eat sporadically and/or automatically. Do not prepare or serve more than can be eaten. Those who are successful with their programs prepare in advance for well balanced meals at home and for upcoming events, even taking their own food to a function if necessary. Always arrange a schedule so that you have time for your exercise sessions and meals. These are two of the most important events of the day. Never skip meals, especially breakfast.
- *Set challenging but realistic goals.* Goal-oriented people are usually successful with most of their efforts. However, you must be realistic with your goals, not to lose too much weight in too short a period of time and

not to have a goal for weight that is most unrealistic for your height and body type. A healthy weight loss rate is no more than two pounds per week.

- *Prepare wisely.* Prepare healthfully by boiling, baking, and steaming. It is very important to include at least 20 percent fat in your meals but be sure that you are getting the proper amount and the healthy fats (see the following 21-Day Detoxification Program).
- *Keep busy and productive.* Do not use eating to occupy leisure time. Always eat the four to five meals per day, but do not break your rule and use eating to occupy leisure time. Be sure that you're exercising regularly, getting the proper kinds of exercise every day. Keeping your body moving continuously raises and keeps your metabolic rate up, burning calories all day, even hours after your exercise session and even when you are resting. The regular exercise will increase your lean body tissue and decrease your body fat tissue, and this raises your metabolic rate in that lean tissue requires calories whereas fat does not.
- *Beware of social binges.* Eat wisely at functions and avoid refrigerator raids. If you use alcohol at all, and especially at social functions, be sure that it's used in great moderation. This is very important to your weight maintenance program and most vital to your healing process from your fibromyalgia.
- *Monitor progress and reward accomplishments.* Keep track of percent body fat and loss in inches and pounds during reasonable periods. Do not be concerned with weighing and measuring on a daily basis. Remember that people who are successful at losing and maintaining their weight and improving their health do not follow stringent or crash diets nor do they burden themselves with calorie counting. Focus on total health and wellness and getting well. Do not be so concerned with numbers on the

scale nor how much farther you can walk each day. Simply allow those things to happen naturally as you are getting healthier, feeling better, and getting well.

- *Practice effective stress management techniques.* Learn deep breathing and muscle relaxation exercises. If you need, go to a professional to learn these procedures in a very efficient manner. Be organized and efficient with time, as this is one of the major stress relievers. Remember to get 7-8 hours of sleep every night, always retiring at the same time establishing a habit pattern to enhance the effective and efficient sleep pattern. Include a minimum of two and possibly three fifteen-minute relaxation sessions on a daily basis. This will add tremendously to your health and vitality and to your recovery.
- *Develop a positive success attitude.* Concentrate on succeeding and not negative past habit patterns or failure. Avoid negative environments and negative people who will not be supportive. Focus on why you have developed poor eating habits and what those poor habits were, times of day you were eating, what you were eating and how you were preparing. Finally, make a conscious effort to change those behaviors.

DR. ELROD'S 21-DAY DETOXIFICATION PROGRAM

Detoxification is the process of body and/or cell cleansing through purging of toxic buildup resultant of a combination of poor diet, ingestion of abusive substances, and stress. An abusive lifestyle, including the ingestion of excessive fat, junk foods, nicotine, caffeine, excessive alcohol, other drugs, a lack of rest, and undue stress will eventually create a toxic buildup within the body and begin to break down the immune system.

10-day Tapering period

I have designed the following dietary guidelines to promote body cleansing as a first step back toward health and wellness, and as a new beginning for strengthening the immune system. The body doesn't like shock, so ideally a ten-day tapering period of gradually reducing sugar, fat, caffeine, etc., is advised before beginning the 21-day detoxification program. The ten-day tapering period is important in assisting the body to adjust and to ensure success with the total program. As you can see, within a 30-day period, the cleansing (detoxification) process will be complete and you will be on your way back to a happy, healthy, and successful lifestyle.

Things to Emphasize

These are areas that one should emphasize in nutritional habits for achieving a successful detoxification program:

1. Eat 5 or 6 small meals throughout the day.
2. Increase high fiber foods, gradually: vegetables, fresh fruits, whole grains, seeds and nuts, and legumes. Be sure to include peaches, strawberries, potatoes, spinach, tomatoes, wheat and bran cereals, whole wheat bread, rice, and popcorn.
3. Increase raw fruits and vegetables to 50 percent of your diet. Be sure to include cucumbers, radishes, grapefruit, apples, carrots, cantaloupe, red bell peppers, and green leafy vegetables.
4. Drink pure water (10 to 12 glasses a day).
5. Eat moderately and more deliberately. No television or reading while eating; emphasize family conversation.
6. Eat a maximum of 1500 calories per day for 21 days.
7. Employ the thankful heart attitude for your food and health.

8. Visualization: For each of these 21 days, visualize yourself getting well while maintaining your ideal body weight and shape.

Things to Avoid

The following are foods and other nutritional to avoid in order to achieve a successful detoxification program:

1. High fat dairy products
2. White sugar and white flour
3. Fried foods
4. Preservatives, junk food, and salt
5. Red meat (especially salt-cured, smoked, nitrate-cured foods like bacon, pepperoni, etc.) and chicken (which is a high-fat food)
6. Coffee and caffeinated teas
7. Colas, soda pop, and carbonated beverages
8. Liquids with your meals (Drink acceptable liquids one hour before and two hours after meals. Drinking during meals dilutes hydrochloric acid.)
9. Alcoholic beverages
10. All forms of tobacco
11. Prolonged periods in direct sun rays (Protect yourself with at least 15 spf sunscreen; wear long sleeves and hat between 11 a.m. and 3 p.m.)
12. NutraSweet and saccharine.

Note: Consume 25 percent of total calories at breakfast. Consume 50 percent of total calories at lunch. Consume 25 percent of total calories at dinner. (Do not count the two or three healthful snacks.)

NOW WHAT AFTER 21 DAYS?

After you have successfully completed your detoxification and immune system strengthening program, you will not necessarily continue with the above stringent nutritional program. However, you will want to continue a prudent, healthful program to keep you on track for a happy, healthy, successful life. For example, you will want to adhere to the following healthful eating guidelines:

- Remember to continue the habit pattern of eating 5-6 small meals throughout the day.
- Continue high fiber content in diet (fruits, vegetables, whole grains and cereals).
- Choose whole wheat breads, bran cereals, rice, and pasta.
- Consume legumes (beans, lentils and nuts).
- Use low-fat dairy products.
- Limit or eliminate red meats.
- Eat chicken or turkey (no skin), tuna and fish in place of red meat.
- Emphasize fruits, vegetables, and salads (low-cal dressings).
- Ingest omega-3 fatty acids (fish oils).
- Drink purified water (10 to 12 glasses per day).
- Increase calories back to normal maintenance levels for active individuals (1800 to 2400 for females, 2400 to 3000 for males) once desired weight has been achieved.

Problems with Additives, Metals and Other Toxins

There is a strong link between heavy toxic metals, food additives, other toxins and poor nutrition. Toxic metals are commonly found in commercially processed foods that typically contain food colorings and additives. Pesticides, herbicides and other agricultural chemicals still present us with numerous nutritional issues. The following sections address the problems with metals, food additives and other toxins commonly consumed in the average diet (For more complete information on this topic, see Dr. Skye Weintraub's title, Natural Treatments for ADD and Hyperactivity, 1997).

METALS

Let's take a loo k at some of the metals commonly found in the body and that become toxic and cause degenerative and serious health problems. There are treatment plans available for treating and removing toxic metals from the body and there are also naturopathic health practitioners who do toxicity testing.

Mercury

Mercury amalgam tooth fillings are one of the primary sources for mercury leakage into the body. Some of the other common places to find mercury include processed foods, drinking water, pesticides, fertilizers, mascara, floor waxes, body powder, adhesives, wood preservatives, batteries, and air conditioning filters. Finally, mercury is second only to cadmium as being the most toxic heavy metal on earth.

Lead

Lead is linked to a number of neurological and psychological disturbances. Lead affects brain function because of its neurotoxic effects. Our drinking water appears to be one of the more prominent sources from which we accumulate lead into the body.

One precaution is to have your water supply tested for high lead levels. The use of lead-based solders in modern copper plumbing systems increases the intake of lead through the very water we drink. Filter your home water supply with a filter that will remove heavy metals.

Always wash your fruits and vegetables in filtered water before use, not tap water. If possible buy your produce from farms and areas that have low air pollution. Do not use any imported canned food as the cans are often lead lined.

Copper

Stress from fibromyalgia can lead to copper toxicity. When the adrenal glands function properly, they produce a copper bonding protein, therefore, stress can deplete zinc from body tissue which taxes the adrenal glands. People who consume large amounts of soda pop, junk foods, and other empty-calorie foods are much more prone to copper toxicity problems. This can help to lower the immune system and cause the individual to have recurrent infections more readily.

Manganese

Excessive toxic levels of manganese are toxic to the brain's neurons. There is typically emotional instability associated with manganese overload, such as easy laughter or crying, muscular weakness, slowed speech, and impaired equilibrium.

Cadmium

Cadmium levels are typically higher in people that eat excessive amounts of carbohydrates. This suggests that the consumption of fast or refined foods that are low in nutrients increases the body's cadmium levels. Adequate zinc intake may help protect against the adverse effects of cadmium. Once cadmium is in the body it is very difficult to remove because of its seventeen to thirty year life span. Elimination of cadmium from the body is generally accomplished through nutritional therapy (See the 21-day Detoxification Program).

Cigarettes are one of the major sources of cadmium in our society. Zinc, used for galvanizing iron, can contain up to two percent cadmium and this is one reason our tap water is normally contaminated.

Aluminum

High levels of aluminum affect the central nervous system and is suspected to be intricately involved in the problems of fibromyalgia sufferers. Some of the primary sources of aluminum are in the very aluminum cookware used in homes, as well as aluminum foil in which we frequently store food. Aluminum is also found in antacids, bleached flour, and coffee. Deficiencies of magnesium and calcium may greatly increase the toxic effects of aluminum in the body.

FOOD ADDITIVES TO AVOID

About 70-80 percent of the foods we consume undergo some degree of refinement or chemical alteration. The Department of National Health and Welfare explains that additives are usually chemical in nature and do not include seasonings, spices, or natural flavorings. Consumers in

America use approximately 100 million pounds of food additives per year. The FDA in the United States allows more than 10,000 food and chemical additives in our food supply. The average American consumes between 10 and 15 pounds of salt and additives per year (Gans, 1991).

There are two categories of food additives: those that make food more pleasant to the eyes and more appealing to the taste buds and, secondly, those that prevent food from spoiling or that increase their shelf life.

BHT

Butylated hydroxytoluene (BHT) retards rancidity in frozen and fresh pork sausage and freeze-dried meats. The base product used in shortenings and animal fats contains BHT and is also the base product for chewing gum. Enlargement of the liver and allergic reactions are two of the adverse effects that have been exhibited from the use of BHT.

BHA

Butylated hydroxyanisole (BHA) is also an antioxidant and effects liver and kidney function within human beings. BHA has been associated with behavior problems in children and is commonly used as a preservative in a wide variety of products like baked goods, candy, chewing gum, soup bases, breakfast cereals, shórtening, dry mixes for desserts, potatoes, potato flakes, and ice cream.

Caffeine

Caffeine can affect blood sugar release and uptake by the liver and is a central nervous system, heart, and respiratory stimulant. Caffeine is a natural ingredient in tea, coffee, and cola and some of its ill effects are irregular heartbeat, ear noises, insomnia, irritability and nervousness.

Aspartame

Equal and NutraSweet are the actual marketed names of aspartame. Aspartame intensifies the taste of sweeteners and flavors and is about 200 times sweeter than sucrose. Recent research studies have discovered that memory loss attributed to diabetes is caused by aspartame. Large amounts consumed over time will upset neurotransmitter balance as well as the amino acid balance within the body.

MSG

Canned tuna, snack foods, and soups and a large percentage of prepared foods now found on grocery store shelves contain MSG. Monosodium glutamate is now the most common flavor enhancer added to foods on the market.

It is very difficult to identify MSG within products from labels because the manufacturers are not required to call it MSG on the label. MSG is very frequently disguised with such names as sodium caseinate, hydrolyzed yeast, hydrolyzed vegetable protein, and autolyzed yeast. Some of the other names used to disguise MSG are textured protein, hydrolyzed protein, yeast food, calcium caseinate, natural chicken or turkey flavoring, yeast extract, hydrolyzed yeast, natural flavoring, and other spices.

Phosphates

Phosphates attract the trace minerals in foods and then continue to remove them from the body. There are phosphates in cheese, baked goods, carbonated drinks, canned meats, powdered foods, dry cereals, and cola drinks. Phosphates are a preservative that prevent the outward and chemical changes of food including texture, appearance, flavor, and color.

Sorbate

Sorbate is a fungus preventative and preservative used in chocolate syrups, drinks, soda fountain syrups, baked goods, deli salads, cheese cake, fresh fruit cocktail, pie fillings, preserves, and artificially sweetened jellies.

Sulfites

Sulfites are preservatives and bleaching agents found in sliced fruit, beer, ale, and wine. They are commonly found in packaged lemon juice, potatoes, salad dressings, gravies, corn syrup, wine vinegar, avocado dip, and sauces.

Sulfites are primarily used to reduce or prevent discoloration of light colored vegetables and fruits such as dehydrated potatoes and dried apples. Sulfites assist vegetables and fruits to look fresh.

Flours and Grains

Grains have been around almost since the beginning of time. Many of our grains are some of the same grains used by the original colonists of the United States, although the processing of these grains have made baking and cooking with them quite different from the times of early settlers. As one becomes more knowledgeable about the different grains, it becomes obvious why the grains were and continue to be such an important part of daily diets. In getting well and maintaining a healthy body it has been very important for me to omit processed white flours from my diet. The next few pages will tell about many of the grains that have replaced white processed flour in our cupboards. Most of these grains can be found in local health food stores, and if they are not available, the stores will know how and where to source them.

Knowing and understanding the different forms of flours and how they work has been helpful in baking with them since baking with flours other than processed white flours can change the size and texture of products baked. To begin, lets take a look at refined white flour. During the process of refining the wheat to create the white flour we know so well and use in the majority of our baking, wheat looses up to 80% of its nutrients. Enriched white flour has only four of the twenty nutrients put back into the flour, making it sixteen nutrients short of what Mother Nature intended. During the process of bleaching the flour, essential amino acid or the protein part of the flour has also been destroyed.

Some flours also contain gluten or protein that controls the bread's ability to raise. Gluten containing grains in descending order are wheat, spelt, Kamut, rye, oats and barley. According to the Rodale Research Center in eastern Pennsylvania, all grains contain some gluten, although those with a very low amount of gluten are considered gluten free. Gluten free grains and non grains are corn, millet, buckwheat, amaranth, quinoa, rice, sorghum and teff.

Grains and flours can become rancid if kept in improper temperatures. To avoid this from happening, it is helpful when buying flours in bulk to store them in the freezer in glass jars and allow the flour to come to room temperature for best results in baking.

TYPES OF GRAINS AND FLOURS

Kamut

Kamut, which originated from the Nile region of Egypt and has never been crossbred. The Kamut grain contains more protein, lipids and measures higher in 88 percent more minerals than found in the common wheat. Kamut wheat contains gluten so if a person is sensitive to gluten, this would be a grain/flour to avoid. Many times those who are sensitive to wheat find Kamut flour to be a good substitute. Kamut has a buttery taste and is much higher in nutritional value than most other grains, containing approximately 30% more protein than other wheats. It is also much higher in amino acids and fatty acids. Kamut flour can be used for almost any baking needs you would use wheat flour in, although, due to its color, baked goods generally will come out browner. For measurements to substitute Kamut wheat for whole wheat flour, see the "Substitution" section in this book.

Spelt

Spelt grain is easily digested, therefore it may be a good grain for those of us who suffer with digestive disturbances. Originating in Asia, spelt contains many of the nutrients and amino acids necessary for a healthy body, therefore it is a grain that is good to keep around for baking needs. This grain, which is very disease resistant has its own protective covering called a husk or hull, which guards the spelt grain against outside pollutants. This protective husk which must be removed before the grain can be used, protects the spelt grain during the growing process and in storage. Although the spelt grain has more of a buttery flavor than the wheat grain, it can be used in place of wheat flour in cooking and baking. I have found spelt as a great flour substitute for white processed flours, using it in most of the recipes that call for white processed flour. The baked goods come out with similar consistency as they would with processed flour, although many times the buttery flavor can be noticed adding a wonderful addition to baked goods.

Oat

For those who have high cholesterol or high blood sugar, oat flour can be a very healthy substitute for wheat flour. It has been found oats help to lower cholesterol, regulate blood sugar, reduce chances of getting certain cancers and push poisonous wastes through your system fast. Oats are a highly nutritious grain that is low in saturated fat, low in cholesterol and has been found to help reduce the risk of heart disease. It is a grain that grows on a stalk similar to the wheat grain. Oat flour seems to add more moisture to cakes and breads, making it "heavier" lthough healthier than wheat. If this flour is difficult to find in your area, it can be made by putting "rolled oats" into a blender and blending until it is of "flour consistency."

Amaranth

Amaranth originated in the Aztecs in Mexico and South America as well as in China and was once considered to be a very important grain and daily staple for health. Today it can be grown in Midwestern states such as Kansas and Nebraska. The seeds of the amaranth plant can be eaten cooked or ground into flour for baking uses. This source of flour is very nutritious as it is a high source of vegetable protein, amino acids, lysine, vitamins and minerals. Due to the lack of gluten in amaranth flour, a gluten product such as potato starch, corn starch, tapioca starch or soy flour needs to be added in many recipes. This gluten-free plant is related to the pigweed family so in many cases can be used as a substitute by those who are allergic to grains. Once purchased, this grain is best stored in the freezer. If not stored properly this flour can develop a strong odor, become rancid or bitter.

Barley

Barley is a cereal grass native to Asia and Ethiopia. Its leaves have become a popular source of the antioxidant and phytochemical properties recommended by natural healers. Barley contains a large proportion of carbohydrates and protein and was used to help conserve wheat by replacing part of the wheat flour in recipes with barley flour. Barley flour has a strong flavor so generally would be used with another grain in baking.

Buckwheat

Buckwheat is a grain that has the highest source of protein in the plant kingdom, higher than that of soybeans. In comparing the protein content in buckwheat to that of beef, in poundage, twice the weight of buckwheat can provide the same amount of protein as in half the same weight in beef. The amino acids found in buckwheat, allows the protein in it to be used by our bodies in the most efficient way possible. It is native of shores on the Caspian Sea and was introduced into western Europe during the 16th century. The seeds that are ground into flour are tiny black, three cornered seeds. The buckwheat plant is actually a fruit since it has seeds and is closely related to the rhubarb plant. It is grown organically and is a great source for vitamins, minerals and dietary fiber, and has been found to be helpful in preventing atherosclerosis. It is a fat and cholesterol free food. Twenty percent of our suggested daily fiber intake can be found in one cup of ground buckwheat. Buckwheat can be used as a flour in griddle cakes and some breads or it can be eaten as a cooked cereal.

Corn

Corn flour is made from whole kernels of corn that are finely ground. This flour comes in white or yellow depending on the color of corn used to make the flour. It is used in combination with other flours in baked goods or is used for breading for meats or vegetables. The basic ingredient for corn tortillas is Masa Harina, which is a special type of corn flour. Cornstarch is obtained from the part of the kernel called the endosperm. Corn is a gluten-containing corn, so should be avoided when a person is gluten intolerant.

Quinoa

Quinoa has been grown in the South American Andes since at least 3,000 B.C. Ancient Inca Indians revered it as a "sacred" grain, and today's research has suggested this grain comes as close to essential life sustaining nutrients of any other in the vegetable or animal kingdoms. There are about 2,000 varieties of Quinoa with colors ranging from off-white to black. It is high in protein, vitamins E and B, and is high in calcium, phosphorous and iron. The bitter coating on the seeds called Saponin, act as a natural insect and bird repellent. This coating forms a soapy solution in water and seeds must be washed two or three times before eating the seed to remove the bitter taste it produces. This seed which is high in oil and fat, can be cooked very quickly for a fast, hot cereal, or the flour can be made into muffins or pancakes.

Rice

Rice is a grain found in the grass family and is gluten free. Due to its popularity, it is the second most produced food in the world and comes in many varieties. It is a natural source of vitamin b, and although it originated in Southeast Asia, China and India, can be found growing around the world including countries such as South America, United States, China, Africa, Australia, India, Italy, Spain and Asia. Rice flour has a dryer consistency and leaves a "grainier" taste when used in cooking. It is a very good alternative flour to be used in place of other white or brown flours. There are a number of varieties such as brown rice, sweet brown rice, Basmati, Texmati, Calmati and other "specialty" forms.

Soy

Soy flour is made from soy beans that have been roasted and ground into a powder and has a long shelf life of up to twelve months. It can be found in either full-fat which contains the natural oils found in the soy bean or low-fat which has the oils removed. It is an excellent source of protein, iron vitamin-B and calcium and isoflavones which can help prevent certain chronic diseases such as cancer, heart disease and osteoporosis. Low-fat soy flour is also a good source of fiber. Eggs can be substituted in a recipe by replacing one egg with one tablespoon soy flour and one tablespoon water. Products baked with soy flour may brown sooner, so the oven temperature should be lowered slightly during baking. It should be stirred before measuring it since it tends to pack down in the container.

REFINED FLOURS

Refined flours made from wheat

Refined flours may carry a number of different names including All-Purpose Flour, Bread Flour, Self-Rising Flour, Cake Flour and Pastry Flour. To better understand these flours and the differences that occur during processing let's take a look at the nutritional content of whole grains versus their refined flours.

Calorie content of refined flour made from wheat actually increases about ten percent because everything else has been taken out. Approximately sixty six percent of the B vitamins, seventy percent of all minerals and an average of nineteen percent of protein has been removed. Fiber content has decreased about seventy nine percent. Except for the carbohydrates, most nutritional value has been removed from refined flours.

Let's take a look at those flours that have been fortified with vitamins and their nutritional content. Two nutrients that have been removed during processing, vitamins B6 and folacin, are not replaced. Of the nine minerals removed from processed flours, only three, calcium, phosphorus and iron are sometimes replaced in fortified flours. Be sure to check the label to be sure at least these three have been fortified in the flour. Many of the vitamins and minerals that are replaced in processed, fortified flours, have undergone a processing that leaves them in a state in which our digestive systems have a very low absorption rate. When we eat refined flours, we are eating a very nutrient poor food, far from the wheat and its nutrients intended by Mother Nature.

Refined meals made from corn

During its refinement process, cornmeal loses much less of its nutritional content than wheat flours, since its refinement process is much less. It isn't harmed significantly by the refinement process, although the biggest drawback is the oils becoming rancid if the meal isn't freshly ground making them less nutritious. Grinding fresh corn for corn meal is delicious compared to cornmeal found on grocery shelves.

Buckwheat flour does not seem to be significantly harmed by refinement retaining approximately eighty five to one hundred percent of its nutrients.

SUBSTITUTIONS

We will begin this section of the book with substitutions for wheat. To have a smoother texture when baking with rice flour, the Rice Council of America also suggests to: Mix the rice flour with the liquid called for in a recipe. Bring to a boil, then cool before adding other ingredients.

Also, according to the Rice Council of America coarse flours don't need to be sifted before measuring, however, they need more leavening than wheat flour. For each cup of coarse flour, use 2 1/2 tsp. of baking powder.

These substitutions are recommended by the Rice Council of America.

For 1 cup of wheat flour substitute:
3/4 c. sweet rice flour
1 scant c. corn meal (fine)
1 c. corn flour
5/8 c. potato starch flour
3/4 c. corn meal

These are other wheat flour substitutes. For 1 cup of wheat flour, substitute the following:
1 c. amaranth flour 1 c. millet flour
1 1/3 c. oat flour
1 1/4 c. rye flour
7/8 c. kamut flour
1 c. spelt flour
7/8 c. buckwheat flour
1 1/3 c. barley flour
3/4 c. garbanzo bean (chickpea) or other bean flours
1 c. quinoa
1/2 c. soy +1/2 c. potato starch

Substitutes for 1 c. whole-wheat flour include:
1 c. kamut flour
1 c. spelt flour (reduce the amount of liquid by 25 percent)

To replace 1 T. of Wheat flour as a thickener use:
1 1/2 tsp. Arrowroot   1 1/2 tsp. cornstarch
1 Tbsp. oat flour   2 tsp. tapioca
1 Tbsp. brown or white rice flour

Sweeteners

Since eliminating sugars playes such a vital role in regaining my health it was important to learn more about sweeteners available in our markets. Studies have showm each person eats between 35 and 150 teaspoons of sugar per day, which adds up to 65 to 150 pounds (cane or beet) sugar and 79 pounds of corn sweeteners per year. Since sugar provides "empty" calories, it is not suprising that many Americans have problems with obesity. Another suprising statistic is the 16 pounds of artificial or chemical sweeteners consumed by Americans each year. Sweeteners may be the cause of health problems ranging from kidney damage to allergies to cancer. Sugars have no fiber or nutrition!

The more "natural" sweeteners may seem to contain more vitamins and minerals, although, through commercial processing these sweeteners can lose much of their vitamin content. For instance, commercially processed, honeys may lose between 33% to 50% of their original vitamin content.

SWEETENERS, WHAT ARE THEY?

Glucose is sometimes called dextrose or blood sugar. Fructose is found naturally in fruits and honey and is a simple sugar. Lactose comes from milk, better known as "milk sugar. Sucrose is a mixture of fructose and glucose. Maltose occurs naturally in sprouted grain. Let's take a look at a number of sugars:

Brown Rice Syrup: Brown rice syrup is made from slow cooking brown rice until it develops into a thick, sweet syrup. It has been a traditional Asian sweetener for many years and is considered to be a complex sugar. It is interchangeable with honey in cooking and baking.

Barley Malt: Barley Malt syrup is milder than blackstrap molasses and not as sweet as honey. This syrup enters the bloodstream slowly and offers trace amounts of B vitamins and several minerals. This sweetener is made from sprouted, roasted barley grain and has a sweet, nutty flavor. It comes in granular form or syrup.

Fructose: Fructose is the sugar derived from fruit, and closely resembles white sugar. It is twice as sweet as white sugar, so 1/2 as much can be used as white sugar. It breaks down more slowly in the body than sugar and does not provide any nutritional benefits.

Date Sugar: Date sugar is made from ground, dehydrated dates, therefore, it is actually not a sugar. It is high in vitamins and minerals and has a high concentration of naturally occuring sugars. This sugar doesn't dissolve well but is good for cooking and baking.

Fruit Juice Sweetener: This sweetener goes through very little processing and is generally made from juices of pineapple, pear, peach or clarified grape juice.

Honey: Honey is primarily glucose, a simple sugar. Commercially processed, clarified honey looses from 33% to 50% of its original vitamin content. Raw honey contains one of the highest enzyme contents of all foods, and in its raw state has many minerals. The flavor of honey varies with the flower used to make it. Some of the types of honey one might find on the store shelves would be buckwheat, clover, orange blossom, wildflower and sage. Each has a flavor all its own, and is delicious to use in many ways.

Maple Syrup: This syrup is made from boiling dowm the sap from the maple tree, and is mainly sucrose, a simple sugar. Maple syrup is classified in grade by its color, the lighter the color, the lighter the flavor. Maple syrup is not good for pancakes, but adds a wonderful flavor to baked goods.

Molasses: Molasses is formed from the liquid spun out of cane sugar during processing. It is graded by color and consits of 20-25% water, 50% sucrose, and 10% ash, and includes some protein and organic acids. It is rich in iron and vitamin B6, calcium and potassium. Organic, unsulphured molasses is best for optimal quality.

Sorghum: Sorghum, a grain related to millet, is processed into a sweetener by crushing the stocks and boiling the extracted juice into a syrup. It is lighter and milder than molasses.

Sucanat: Sucanat, contains more vitamins, minerals and other trace nutrients than sugar cane. It is made from the dehydrated juice of the organic sugar cane, and is about 88% sucrose or simple sugar, as compared to table sugar, which is 99% sucrose. It has a flavor that is similar to a very mild molasses flavor and can be used in most cooking and baking.

Stevia: Stevia comes from an herb and is about 10-15 times sweeter than regular sugar. This wonderful sweetener contains nearly one hundred identified phytonutrients and volatile oils. Since stevia is much sweeter than sugar, the amounts consumed to sweeten food make the nutritive benefits very little. Research has shown stevia may actually lower blood sugar levels, making it a natural substitute, that can be used by diabetics. For many years, stevia has been grown overseas, and in the past few years it has been grown in gardens in the United States, making it a very accessible and inexpensive sweetener to have in ones cupboards.

Turbinado: Turbinado comes from molasses during the first separation in processing. It is identical to white sugar in the way it is absorbed.

In working towards eliminating sugars from the diet, the following chart may be helpful in making substitutions. These measurements are equal to 1 cup of sugar:

SWEETENER	SOURCE	TO REPLACE 1 C SUGAR	LIQUID REDUCTION
Brown Rice Syrup	brown rice	1 cup	1/4 cup
Fructose	corn or beet	1/2 cup	3/4 cup
Date Sugar	dates	2/3 cup	----
Barley Malt	barley	1 cup	1/4 cup
Fruit Juice	fruit	1 cup	1/8 cup
Honey	bees	1/2 cup	1/4 cup
Maple Syrup	maple trees	1/2-1/3 cup	----
Molasses	sugar cane	1/2 cup	1/4 cup
Sorghum	sorghum	1/2 cup	1/4 cup
Sucanat	organic cane	1 cup	----
Stevia	herb	1-1/1/2 TBSP	----
Turbinado	sugar cane	1 cup	----

Herbs

One of the areas of cooking I have found to be most rewarding as well as enjoyable is using and cooking with herbs. As far back as time the garden has been given an image of a wellspring of spiritual and physical healing. Realizing the garden has been with us since the very early years of mankind lends a richness and depth to our connection of gardens. The garden brings with it a peacefulness that may be difficult to find in a world of deadlines and hurry. Once established, a garden can be a refuge from life itself, bringing smells and beauty unsurpassed by any other. It's healing plants can become a focal point for health, adding flavor and nourishment to the very food we eat to replenish our bodies.

Not only are herbs full of vitamins and minerals, they help create new and exciting flavors in most dishes they are used in. For the avid or novice gardener, herbs can bring an array of color to the yard as most of them bloom for weeks during the warmer months. From June until the end of September my garden is a shower of color ranging from yellows to purples to blues and pinks. Flowers to set on my kitchen table are in abundance during the summer months, and each herb has an aroma that fills my home with the pleasant smells of the best nature has to offer. My personal favorite is basil, as it's beautiful blue bell like flowers and wonderful smells can fill a room within minutes of it's arrival. Second in line is Sage. The sage leaf is a soft, silver green, almost like a lambs ear. The purple flowers last only a few days after being cut, although when hung upside down in a darkened room to dry, this plant can be used to create a wonderful display for winter bouquets.

Becoming an advocate for growing herbs in ones own garden came quite by accident for me. In 1990 we moved into a small home in central Missouri. The home had been empty for a short time before we moved into it and the weeds had begun to take over around the house and yard. During the first year after we moved into the home, I tried to get the "weeds" under control. Most of them responded to my pulling and tugging and finally disappeared, although there was one weed that didn't respond like the others. This weed emitted the most aromatic smell when I would try to pull it and the more I pulled it the faster more plants of the same type would come up out of the ground. Finally, out of frustration I called a friend who was fairly knowledgeable about plants and asked her to come to my home and help me figure out what type of a plant this was. Once she arrived, it took her about five seconds of looking at the plant and smelling the leaves before she made the determination this plant was spearmint. She strongly urged me to learn more about it's medicinal uses. Thus began what would become the herbal portion of my healing process from fibromyalgia/chronic fatigue syndrome.

Later that day I ventured to the library and began finding herbal books from which I learned spearmint was very helpful in settling the stomach. As time continued, spearmint also became my "herb of choice" for many maladies including the common stomach flu. As the years have passed, the simple spearmint plant in our garden has been called upon to help with headaches, indigestion, insomnia, sore throats, to help relieve tension and as a gargle for sore throats.

Today, many years later, our yard is my medicine chest, providing relief for many physical maladies as well as seasoning our meals. During the early years of my healing, the herbal garden provided a wonderful distraction from the pain and symptoms that plagued my body. It gave me a "reason" to be outside, which can be so beneficial in the healing process. Today it is the pride and joy of my summers as these very plants that helped promote healing in my body continue to share an abundance of color. And, throughout the summer and in the winter they remind me of their presence by improving flavors in my cooking and helping with other viruses and physical maladies that may come along. Growing herbs is one of the most fulfilling and least expensive hobbies there is. In addition, one of the most wonderful things about growing an herbal garden is the gardener is free to spend five minutes or five hours enjoying this hobby. There are no rules or regulations determining when the "gates" will open since the gates are never closed.

GROWING HERBS

An herbal garden is one of the simplest of gardens to keep, as many of the herbs, if put into ground conducive to their healthy existence, will spread and kill most of the "weeds" that may try to creep in around it.

Growing herbs can be very simple. The soil in our area is a very thick clay type of soil, and is not conducive to growing much of anything other than weeds. The first fall we lived in our home I began collecting leaves that had fallen to the ground and piling them on the area where I intended to begin my garden. Of course if you live in an area where the soil is already very healthy, this step wouldn't be as important, although, the leaves provided more than nitrogen which is so important for healthy plants, it provides a nesting place for lady bugs and other helpful insects.

During the winter months our neighbors provided ashes from their fireplaces onto the area we had planned for our herbal garden. The following spring I tilled the leaves and ashes into the soil, picked out the herbs I wanted to grow that season and planted them into the prepared garden area. Throughout the summer I would catch the grass clippings whenever we mowed and place them around the plants, thus providing more nitrogen and a natural weed barrier. Interesting also, the grass clippings also provided a nesting place for more beneficial bugs as well as bringing a tremendous amount of worms closer to the surface of the ground. The worms are very helpful in cleansing and loosening the soil. Within a few short weeks the herbs began to explode in size and shortly after that began to fill our garden and our homes with color and wonderful aromas.

HARVESTING HERBS

Herbs can be harvested at any time, although there are times during the day and months during which the oils and medicinal properties of the herbs are at their peak. They can be picked at any time for fresh use. There are a few helpful suggestions for harvesting herbs during the times their oils are the strongest. Harvesting before noon assures the volatile oils will be at their peak. Also, the month between full moons is best since moonlight saps their strength. Also, it is important to wait a day or two after a rain to harvest since rain washes away some of the aromatic oils from many herbs.

To harvest, prune the tips of the plant one-fourth to one-third, or culling the whole stocks. Hang upside down in a paper sack that has holes or slits in the side of the sack to allow air circulation. Harvesting is very simple and I have found it generally works best to continue to collect the herbs in bags and store them in a closed, darkened room until fall. Then, in storing the plants for the winter, slide the fingers down the dried stems to remove the leaves. Store in well-sealed jars in a dark, dry, cool place.

FAVORITE HERBS

There are many herbs that have become my favorite to use for healing and for cooking. Many of these herbs are interchangeable in their uses of cooking and healing properties, thereby giving the grower two for one.

MINT
Medicinal Uses: Helps to relieve tension, insomnia, nervousness and trembling.
Cooking Uses: Teas, carrots, peas, potatoes, sweet potatoes, spinach, cabbage, zucchini
Garden Insects It Helps Control: Colorado beetles, ants
Companion Plants: cabbage, plants in general

CATNIP
Medicinal Uses: Calmative, immune system booster, relax intestinal cramping, anxiety and headaches
Cooking Uses: (Never boil or it will lose its medicinal qualities.)
Teas (Use with mint for a wonderful drink)
Garden Insects It Helps Control: Colorado beetles
PARSLEY
Medicinal Uses: High in vitamins and minerals. In the past this plant was used as a diuretic, liver tonic and to help break up kidney stones although too much fresh parsley can irritate the kidneys. A poultice made from parsley can be applied to help relieve insect bites. Parsley can help freshen the breath and neutralize garlic odor after eating fresh garlic.
Cooking Uses: Creamed vegetables, potatoes, chopped for garnish or sprinkled on top of fish, while it is baking, chicken soups and dishes, stews and stuffings, all eggs, cheese and sauces, omelets and italian sauces
Salads: All vegetable and seafood salads
Good Garden Companions: asparagus, carrot, chive, tomatoes

Garden Insects It Helps Control: Asparagus beetles

BASIL
Medicinal Uses: Helps relieve nausea and headaches, expel gas
Cooking Uses: cabbage, eggplant, onions, creamed potatoes, squash, turnips, bluefish, halibut, mackerel, shrimps, sole, liver, lamb, veal, sausage, meat stews, ham and beef loaf, tomato soup, vegetable soup, turtle soup, minestrone soup, seafood, tomato juice, stuffed celery, cream cheese, omelets, spaghetti, chicken, seafood and pickled beets
Good Companion Plants: bean, cabbage, tomato
Garden Insects It Helps Control: aphids, asparagus, beetle

DILL
Medicinal Uses: Carminative, helpful for lung congestion
Cooking Uses: cabbage, carrots, creamed potatoes, zucchini, any shellfish, lamb, tomato soup, cheese and onion dishes, tomato juice, dilly bread, cheddar cheese, cottage cheese, spanish omelet
Good Companion Plants: cabbage, lettuce, onions
Garden Insects It Helps Control: none

OREGANO
Medicinal Uses: Contains many antioxidants and rosmarinic acid
Cooking Uses: broccoli, cabbage, mushrooms, onions, tomatoes, lentils, use with melted butter in shellfish stuffings, lamb, pork, veal, sausage, meat loaf, ravioli, chili, chicken, stuffings, tomato soup, bean soup, minestrone, vegetable soup, guacamole, tomato juice, any egg dishes, butter sauce, mixed greens, potato, seafood, tomato
Garden Companions: cabbage, cucumber

ROSEMARY

Medicinal Uses: Helpful with depression, headaches, insomnia, and mental fatigue

Cooking Uses: cabbage, green beans, mushroms, cauliflower, spinach, peas, turnips, any shellfish, creamed, meat loaf, ham loaf, roast pork, all stews, lamb, veal ragout, chicken soup, pea soup, spinach soup, turtle soup, fruit cup, creamed cheese, cottage cheese, french dressing, fish sauces, apple sauce, chopped cabbage, fruit, pear, orange, cole slaw

Good Garden Companions: Bean, cabbage, carrot

BAY LEAF

Medicinal Uses: Help with digestion

Cooking Uses: onions, squash, pickled fish, goulash, liver, lamb, beef stews, soup stock, stuffed eggs, any egg or cheese dish, bernaise, tartar, fish, mixed greens, chicken, fish, somato, any salad dressing

SAGE:

Medicinal Uses: (never boil) Increases physical strength, mental equanimity and alertness, and body heat, baths for muscle and joint pain.

Cooking Uses: succotash, beans, limas, eggplant, onions, tomatoes, creamed corn, pork and beans, sauté crab, baked fish, stuffings, baked ham, stews, veal, pork, sausage, stuffings, all poultry, chowders, cream soups, turtle soup, tomato soup, cottage cheese, cheddar cheese, any egg or cheese dish, chicken, cole slaw, cucumber, potato, tomato

Garden Companions: cabbage, carrot, marjoram, strawberry, tomato

Garden Insects It Helps Control: Cabbage worms

TARRAGON

Medicinal Uses: Helps break down meat and proteins, stimulates the appetite, relieves flatulence and colic, regulate menstruation, alleviate the pain of arthritis, rheumatism and gout, expels worms from the body

Cooking Uses: mushrooms, asparagus, beets, green beans, peas, tomato, celery, baked potatoes, any fish or shellfish, veal, roast beef, sweetbreads, steaks, chops, chicken, game, turkey, duck, consommé chicken, tomato soup, vegetable soup, mushroom soup, spinach soup, fish cocktail, tomato juice, cheese spread, eggs creole, spaghetti sauce, seafood, tomato-aspic

THYME

Medicinal Uses: Alleviate Asthma, Stomach Cramps, whooping cough

Cooking Uses: beets, carrots, onions, peas, mushrooms, rice, stuffed peppers, eggplant, broiled, baked, fried fish, shrimp, oysters, codfish, veal, pork, roast, meat loaf, chicken, stuffings, clam chowder, borscht, tomato soup, pea soup, black bean soup, oyster stew, fish cocktail, clam juice, tomato juice, cheese on crackers, scrambled eggs and omelets, any cheese, macaroni, butter for fish, tomato, mixed greens, seafood, vegetables

Good Garden Companions: Cabbage, plants in general

Garden Insects It Helps Control: Cabbage worms

CILANTRO (coriander)

Medicinal Uses: Flatulence, bloating and cramps, counters nervous tension, if chewed, helps sweeten the breath

Cooking Uses: carrots, potatoes, celery, onions, peas, stuffed peppers, corn, tomatoes, sprinkle on baked fish, chicken, beef, beef roast, Mexican dishes, chicken soup, cheese, guacamole, salsas, cheese spreads, cheddar cheese, cottage cheese

Good Companion Plants: Anise, Potato
Garden Insects It Helps Control: Aphids, spider mites

MUSTARD
Medicinal Uses: headaches, aid digestion or stimulate appetite
Cooking Uses: cabbage, vegetable relishes, potatoes, shrimp, crabs, any other type of fish, ham, chicken, beef

Beginning Changes in Eating Habits

Have healthy food available in your home so you can "snack" any time of the day. Munching on something healthy such as couple of small slices of apple, orange or other fruit or drinking 1/4 cup of 100 percent fresh fruit juice every 2–3 hours can help with hypoglycemia. Carrot sticks, celery and other already cut foods also work nicely for those quick snacks. If you go out to eat, try to eat out only one meal per day since many times restaurants put chemicals on foods to keep them fresh. Sometimes these chemicals can wreak havoc with already stressed immune systems. You won't know until you're well which restaurants use preservatives that may upset you.

In purchasing foods watch for MSGs or other preservatives. Always try to purchase foods that are as close to nature as possible. To sweeten foods, use a product called "stevia." I use the liquid form. Ten drops of stevia equals one cup of white sugar. You can use as much stevia as you like since it doesn't affect FMS/CF. If you have a difficult time staying away from the white sugar at first, use fructose (fruit sugar), and use only half as much as you would white sugar. The goal is to get completely away from any forms of sugar other than sugars that are actually in the fruits, or to use stevia.

It has been important in our household to schedule our meals for the week in advance. By doing this, I can make a grocery list and purchase the foods needed for those meals. I have found this helps with the grocery bill and keeps from having more fresh produce around than we can eat before it spoils. Each day we can choose from the weekly menu the desired menu for the day.

Many of the recipes can be doubled and frozen, making quick, delicious meals for another time. This helps when time for preparing a meal may be limited. The effort it takes to double a recipe is minimal and can be a big help later when time is limited to prepare a meal.

Have fun preparing and eating the following recipes and know you are working towards a healthier you!

WEEKLY MENU PLAN

Day 1

Breakfast: Rich Fruit Shake (Drinks Section), 1 Breakfast Muffin (Breads Section)

Snack: 1/4 cup nuts or nut mix

Lunch: Tortilla Sandwich (soft taco shell, spread with fat free cream cheese, layered with spinach, shredded carrots and other favorite vegetables, then rolled), small bag baked chips

Snack: apple or banana

Dinner: Meatless Meat Loaf, Baked Potato topped with steamed broccoli and one slice of fat free Swiss Cheese

Bedtime: 1/4 cup apple juice

Day 2

Breakfast: 1 Quick, Easy Egg Tortilla (Main Dishes Section), Cup of herbal tea
Snack: Banana or Orange
Lunch: "Fishless" Fillets sandwich using whole wheat bun, Carrot salad
Snack: 1 Oatmeal cookie or 1/2 cup Fruit Freeze (Desserts Section)
Dinner: Italian Casserole, Yeast Bread
Bedtime: 1/4 apple

Day 3

Breakfast: Bowl of 12 grain cereal, juice or rice/soy milk
Snack: fruit
Lunch: Wheat Biscuits, 4 bean salad, Apple mint drink
Snack: Carrots, Celery and fat free dip
Dinner: Delicious Burritos, Lettuce Salad, , Mixed fruit dish

Day 4

Breakfast: One Breakfast McMuffin (main dishes and soup), glass of fruit juice
Snack: fruit
Lunch: Rice and spinach salad (main dishes and soup section), tea
Snack: vegetables ans fat free dip
Dinner: BBQ turnovers, broccoli salad
Bedtime Snack: banana

Day 5

Breakfast: easy breakfast drink
Snack: whole wheat Bagel with peanut butter
Lunch: three bean salad, slice of banana bread

Snack: nut mixture
Dinner: Grilled Salmon, steamed peas, baked sweet potato
Bedtime Snack: 1/2 apple

Day 6

Breakfast: Dry oatmeal with bananas, stevia and rice milk
Snack: Dried fruit mix
Lunch: Vegetable burger, fruit dessert salad
Snack: cookie
Dinner: Vegetable soup, cornbread

Day 7

Breakfast: Egg Omelet, juice
Snack: apple
Lunch: Non breaded fish sandwich, lettuce salad, tea
Snack: Nut mixture
Dinner: Mexican Chips (Main Dishes & Soup), Mexican
  Corn Bread, Rhubarb Dessert

PLAN YOUR OWN MENU

Day 1
Breakfast   Lunch   Dinner

Day 2
Breakfast   Lunch   Dinner

Day 3
Breakfast   Lunch   Dinner

Day 4
Breakfast   Lunch   Dinner

Day 5
Breakfast   Lunch   Dinner

Day 6
Breakfast   Lunch   Dinner

Day 7
Breakfast   Lunch   Dinner

SECTION 4

Recipes for Health

As the first section of this book discusses, diet and nutrition habits are of utmost importance in combatting and relieving the symptoms of fibromyalgia. However, after such a discussion, many of you may ask yourself the question, "What exactly can I eat?" and "What are some easy and good tasting recipes that I can eat on a regular basis?" In response to this, we have compiled a number of healthy, easy to prepare, and tasty recipes that will satisfy the dietary needs of most of you. For your convenience and ease of use, we have grouped the recipes into their corresponding areas: for example, "breads," "desserts," " main dishes and soups," etc. When using eggs in these recipes, it may be best to use eggs that come from "range chickens." These may be purchased through your local health food store or through a farmer who grows range chickens. It is our hope that these recipes provide a springboard to improving your dietary habits and ultimately your health.

Breads

ZUCCHINI BREAD
(Recipe submitted by Anna Bell)

3 eggs beaten until foamy
Add 1 c. canal oil (may use applesauce instead)
1 1/3 c. Fructose
1 t. vanilla
2 c. zucchini grated, peel and all
Mix together with egg mixture
Add to above:
3 c. whole wheat flour
2 t. cinnamon
1 t. soda
4 t. baking powder
1 t. nutmeg
(Fold in 1 c. nutmeats:optional)

Pour into 2 greased & floured loaf pans (9x5x3). Bake at 350° for 55-60 minutes.

BLUEBERRY YOGURT MUFFINS
(Recipe submitted by Anna Bell)

2 c. Quaker Oat Bran Hot Cereal, uncooked
3 T. fructose
2 t. baking powder
1 carton (8 oz.) plain low fat yogurt
2 egg whites, slightly beaten
1/4 c. skim milk

1/4 c. honey
2 T. canola oil (may substitute applesauce)
1 t. grated lemon peel
1/2 c. fresh or frozen blueberries

Set oven to 450° before mixing. Mix together all ingredients and fold in blueberries. Fill muffin cup almost full. Bake 18-20 minutes or until golden brown and wooden pick inserted in center comes out clean. Remove from pan. Makes 12 delicious muffins.

SWEET CINNAMON BUTTER

1 stick soft butter
1 1/2 t. cinnamon
15–18 drops stevia

Blend together all three ingredients. Store in the refrigerator. Use on warm breads or pancakes in place of other sugar sweetened toppings.

WHEAT BISCUITS

1 1/2 c. wheat flour
1/2 c. kamut flour
4 t. baking powder
1/2 t. salt
1/3 c. softened butter
3/4 c. water

Mix together dry ingredients, add oil and mix well. Add enough water to make soft dough that is not sticky. Mix just enough to moisten dry ingredients. With hands, pat out dough to 3/4-inch thickness on floured board. Cut and place on oiled baking sheet. Bake 18-20 minutes in a 450° oven.

NUTTY BAKING POWDER BISCUITS

1/4 c. flax seed
1/2 c. kamut flakes
1/2 c. wheat or other flakes
(These can be purchased at a health food store)

Blend in blender until in flour form. Then add:
1 c. oat flour
1/4 t. sea salt
2 t. baking powder

Mix in:
1/4 c. sesame oil until mixture resembles pebble size. Add 3/4 c. water and mix together.

Turn out onto oat floured surface. Roll out to 3/4 inch thickness. Bake 450° until light brown. Approximately 7–10 minutes. A double batch of this can be made and frozen to be heated for each meal.

BREAKFAST MUFFINS

3/4 c. spelt flour
1 1/2 T. baking powder
1 1/2 c. Fiber 1 cereal
3/4 c. unsweetened applesauce
2 eggs
1/2 c. fructose sugar
dash salt

1 T. cinnamon
1/2 t. allspice
3/4 c. milk (soy or rice milk can be substituted)

Mix together and put into greased muffin tins.

Topping
1/4 c. fructose
1/3 c. oatmeal ground for 15 seconds in blender

Mix together and sprinkle on each muffin. Bake 350° for 20-25 minutes. (Yield: 15-18 muffins)

FLAT BREAD
Submitted by Jolene Brown

1 c. whole wheat flour (course)
1 c. oat flour
1 c. cornmeal (course)
1 t. baking soda
Stir dry ingredients together in large mixing bowl.
1/4 c. vegetable oil—cut into dry ingredients
3/4 c. buttermilk and honey to equal 2 T. sugar

Preheat oven to 350°. Stir liquid into the dry/oil mixture until it resembles dough like piecrust. Separate into 3 balls, kneading each ball in hands about 30 seconds each. On lightly floured surface, roll each ball as thinly as possible (like piecrust.) Roll back onto rolling pin and unroll on an ungreased cookie sheet. Price many places with tines of a fork. Bake until crisp and slightly brown around edges. (If edges start to get too brown, break them off and return to oven.) Cool on wire rack. Break into pieces. Great with soups dips and spreads.

YEAST BREAD

3 packets dry yeast
1 T. fructose
1 1/2 c. warm water

Dissolve yeast in water with fructose. Let set until yeast begins to grow. Then add:
1 egg (beaten)
1/2 t. sea salt
3 T. vegetable oil
1 1/2 c. warm soy milk
1/2 c. gluten flour
4-6 c. oat flour

Add all of the above ingredients except oat flour to yeast mixture. Mix well. Begin adding oat flour 1/2 cup at a time, stirring bread after each time of adding flour. When dough gets too thick to stir, pour 2 cups of flour out onto counter or tabletop and pour bread dough onto flour. Knead flour into bread dough until dough is no longer sticky. Flour inside of bowl and place dough back into bowl. Set in warm, draft free area until double in bulk. Punch down and shape into loaf shape. Place into a greased loaf pan. Let rise until double in bulk. Bake in oven 350° until top of loaf is light brown (approximately 35-50 minutes). Take out of the oven and turn out onto a towel. Brush top of loaf with butter. (This bread will be more coarse and will not rise as high as those breads made with white flour.)

BANANA OAT BREAD

2 c. oat flour
1/4 t. sea salt
3/4 c. mashed banana
2 t. baking powder
2 eggs
3 T. cold water
2 T. unrefined vegetable oil
1/2 c. chopped pecans

Grease 8x8 inch pan. Mix dry ingredients. Beat eggs. Add water, oil and mashed bananas. Blend with dry ingredients. Add pecans. Bake 25-30 minutes in an oven heated to 350°.

BAKING POWDER BREAD

1 c. spelt flour
1/2 c. starch
2 1/4 t. baking powder
1/3 t. sea salt
2 T. oil
1 c. water

Preheat oven to 375°. Oil and flour bottom and sides of an 8x8 inch pan. Wisk together dry ingredients. Add water and oil. Mix thoroughly. Transfer batter to pan and spread evenly. Bake for 20 minutes. Bread is done when it sounds hollow when tapped on top surface.

ZUCCHINI PIZZA CRUST

3 c. grated zucchini
1/4 t. sea salt

3 eggs, beaten
1/3 c. rice flour or corn meal
Toppings as desired.

Grate zucchini using a medium grater or the food processor. Press liquid from zucchini. Combine the beaten eggs with rice flour or corn meal, and salt. Mix with the zucchini. Spread evenly over a 9x12 inch baking sheet or 12 inch pizza pan with sides. Bake at 450° for about 12 minutes or till firm. Remove from oven and top as desired. Return to a 350-degree oven and heat until sauce is bubbly and cheese is melted. Serves about 4.

SOUR MILK ROLLS

3/4 c. rice flour
1/2 T. fructose
1/4 c. soy flour
1 egg
1/4 t. baking soda
1/4 c. fat free cottage cheese
2 t. baking powder
1/2 c. sour milk (To make sour milk, add 2 t. vinegar to
     1/2 c. skim milk.)
1/8 t. sea salt
2 T. melted butter

Combine first 6 ingredients. In mixer bowl or blender, place egg, cottage cheese, milk, and melted butter, and blend. Add this to dry ingredients and mix well. Divide and shape into balls and place on a greased cookie sheet. Bake at 350° for 30 minutes.

CORN CHEESE BREAD

1 c. corn
1/3 c. vegetable oil
1 c. corn meal
3/4 c. grated sharp, fat-free cheddar cheese
1/2 t. soda
3 eggs
2 T. butter
1/4 c. skim milk

Preheat oven to 400°. In a mixing bowl, combine the corn, corn meal, eggs, soda, salt and milk. Mix well. Add the shortening and 1/2 c. of cheese. Stir to blend. Melt butter in 9-inch black iron skillet. Place in the oven to heat until butter melts without browning. Pour batter into the skillet. Sprinkle with the remaining cheese and bake for 30 minutes or until the bread is firm and golden brown on top. Yield 8 servings.

BUTTERMILK PANCAKES

2 1/2 c. buttermilk
2 eggs
1/2 t. salt
1 t. baking soda
3 c. spelt flour

Mix buttermilk, eggs, salt, and baking soda thoroughly. Add flour and beat until smooth. Do not over beat. Spoon onto veggie-sprayed hot griddle or pan and cook until top is full of holes and the underside is brown. Turn and brown other side. Batter should be used immediately after mixing.

MEXICAN BREAD

1 lb. can tomatoes, (undrained)
1/4 t. ground cumin
1 (3 1/2 oz.) can chopped green chilies (undrained)
3/4 c. corn meal
1 t. baking powder
2 T. butter or vegetable oil
6 eggs, separated
1/2 t. cream of tartar
1/2 t. salt
1/2 t. crushed oregano
1/4 c. shredded, fat free cheddar cheese

Butter bottom and sides of a 2-quart casserole dish; dust with corn meal. In large saucepan, combine tomatoes, chilies, butter or vegetable oil, salt and the herbs. Cook and stir over medium heat until butter melts. Stir in corn meal and baking powder. Cook, stirring constantly, until mixture thickens, 3-4 minutes. Remove from heat.

In a large bowl, beat egg whites and cream of tarter until stiff but not dry. Separately, beat yolks slightly. Blend a little of corn meal mixture into the yolks; then add remaining cornmeal mixture and stir. Mix with cheese and pour into casserole dish. Bake at 375° for 40 minutes or until an inserted knife comes out clean. Serve at once. Makes 4 servings.

QUICK YEAST ROLLS

1 c. warm water
1 pkg. rapid rise yeast
1 1/2 T. Fructose
2 c. spelt flour

1/4 c. nonfat milk powder.
2 t. vinegar
1 T. skim milk

Combine water, yeast, sugar and allow to sit at room temperature for at least 15 minutes or until foam forms on top of the liquid. Preheat oven to 400°. In large mixing pan combine flour and milk powder. Add vinegar to yeast liquid, stir well and pour into the flour. Mix into a dough ball and knead for 4 or 5 minutes. Sprinkle with more flour to facilitate kneading. Cut into biscuits and place in veggie sprayed 9 inch cake pan. Brush tops with skim milk and sprinkle with cheese. Allow to sit on top of stove for 10 minutes then bake for 20 minutes.

FRENCH TOAST

Use bread that is free of white flour for this recipe.
4 eggs
3 T. milk
1/8 t. salt
1/4 t. cinnamon
2 T. butter

Melt butter in skillet. Beat eggs, milk, salt and cinnamon. Put slice of bread into egg mixture, turn. Put bread/egg mixture into hot skillet and brown on both sides. Serve with cinnamon butter mixture or fruit (blueberries or strawberries are best).

RICE FLOUR BISCUITS

1 c. rice flour
1/3 c. flax seed meal

1/4 c. gluten flour
1/4 c. gluten flour
1/4 c. spelt flour
1/8 c. vegetable oil
1 T. baking powder
1/4 t. soda

Mix dry ingredients together and cut in vegetable oil until crumbly. Add enough water to make a moist fluffy mixture. Drop by spoonfuls onto ungreased baking pan. Bake 350° 7-10 minutes.

RAISIN BISCUITS

2 t. baking pwdr.
2 c. spelt flour
1/2 t. salt
1/4 c. canola oil
1/2 t. cinnamon

Mix together and add:
1 c. cold water
1/2 c. raisins

Roll out onto lightly floured counter until 1/2 to 3/4 inch thick. Cut with glass. Bake 400° until lightly browned.

FRENCH TOAST

1/2 T. butter
1/2 T. olive oil
4 slices whole grain bread
5 eggs
1 T. water

1/4 t. salt
1/8 t. pepper

Heat butter and oil in iron skillet on low. In pie pan mix eggs, water, salt and pepper with mixer. Dip bread slice into egg mixture. When coated, turn bread over and coat other side. Fry in pan until browned on both sides. Top with unsweetened applesauce or fresh fruit.

HOT 7-GRAIN CEREAL

2 c. water
Dash of salt
1/4 c. raisins
1 c. 7-grain cereal

Heat water raisins and salt to boiling. Boil 3-4 minutes. Add cereal and boil another 5 minutes. Remove from heat and add 20 drops stevia and 1/4 t. cinnamon (optional).

SKILLET CORNBREAD

1 large egg
2 c. skim milk
1 c. cornmeal (stone ground)
1/4 c. flax meal
1/2 c. buffalo flour
1 t. olive oil
1 t. baking soda
1 t. baking pwdr.
1/2 t. salt

Heat oven to 450°. Use a 9-10 inch well-seasoned iron skillet. Brush with olive oil around the bottom and sides of pan. Put skillet in the oven as it preheats. Mix together above ingredients. Mix egg into the milk, then mix in flours and flax meal forming a thin batter. When oven has reached 450° and skillet is almost smoking, beat into above batter, soda, salt and baking powder. Pour all at once into the skillet and bake 15 to 20 minutes or until toothpick comes clean after sticking into the center of the bread.

CORNBREAD

3/4 c. cornmeal
1 T. baking powder
1 c. spelt flour or oat flour
3/4 t. salt
2 beaten eggs
1 c. milk
1/4 c. melted butter
1 T. fructose

Preheat oven to 400°. In a medium mixing bowl stir together the flour, sugar, cornmeal, baking powder, and salt. In another bowl combine eggs, milk and melted butter. Add the egg mixture all at once to the dry ingredients. Stir just until moistened. Place in 9x9 inch-greased pan and bake until browned on top and toothpick comes out clean.

7-GRAIN BREAD

(This is very heavy but delicious bread.)
3 pkg. dry yeast
1 1/2 c. warm water
1 t. fructose
1/4 c. soy or rice milk

Dissolve yeast in sugar, water and milk. Add:
1 egg, beaten
1/4 c. flax mill flour
1/2 c. brown rice flour
1 c. 7 grain flour
1/2 t. sea salt

Mix together with yeast mixture. Pour onto approximately 2 c. spelt flour. Knead in the spelt flour adding more flour until dough is pliable and not sticky. Let rise in a warm place 1-hour. Put into a loaf pan and let rise 40 minutes. Bake at 350° until top is brown and loaf sounds hollow when tapped.

Desserts

It is important to remember that even though the desserts on the following pages may be more healthful than recipes you may find in other books, some of them still use fructose. Depending on the person's own body, it may be important to limit desserts eaten with fructose in them to once a week or a couple of times per month. It continues to be important for me to eat "fresh" fruits or fruit mixtures without fructose for the majority of my meals. Listen to your body after you have eaten the dessert. It will tell you if you like me need to drastically "cut" down on "sweets" in your diet. As you understand more how to cook with fruits and stevia, try your own mixes and blends of fruits.

WHIPPED CREAM

1 c. heavy whipping cream
1t. vanilla
1 T. fructose

Use an aluminum bowl that has been in the freezer a few minutes to cool. Whip cream on high until thickened. Add vanilla and fructose. Serve immediately.

CHOCOLATE BANANA CREAM PIE

1 pie crust made from spelt or rice flour or whole wheat
2 c. soy or rice milk
3 eggs
1/4 t. stevia
3 T. carob powder

3 T. cornstarch
1 T. water
1 t. vanilla
2 bananas

Bake crust in a 350° oven until lightly browned. Remove from oven and let cool. Meanwhile, heat milk and carob powder in a heavy saucepan. While milk is heating, separate eggs, To the yolks, add cornstarch and water. Slowly add yolk mixture to hot milk, stirring constantly. Bring up to a boil and boil just for a minute. Add vanilla and cool. Add stevia. Slice bananas into pie shell and pour pudding over them. Beat egg whites until very stiff adding 1/8 t. stevia while beating. Pour over pie and return to the oven until topping is lightly browned.

RAISIN DESSERT

2 c. raisins
1/4 c. date sugar
1/8 c. fructose
1 T. lemon juice
1 c. water
Boil until raisins are tender and add:
1/4 c. water with 1 1/2 T. cornstarch

Cook until thickened. Set aside and mix together:
2 c. rolled oats
7 T. melted butter
1 1/2 T. fructose

Combine melted butter, rolled oats and fructose. Pat 1 1/2 c. of mixture into bottom of a 9x9 inch pan. Pour raisin mixture over mixture on bottom of the pan. Crumble remainder of rolled oat mixture on top. Bake in a 350° oven until raisin mixture is bubbly, approximately 40 minutes.

"NOT-SO-SINFUL" CARROT CAKE

This cake still has a total of 1 1/8 c. of fructose in it, so it should be eaten sparingly.

3/4 c. grape nut cereal
1/8 c. fructose

Mix and sprinkle over bottom of cheesecake pan. Then blend:
2 T. flour
1 egg
1 pkg. fat free cream cheese
1/8 c. fructose
2 T. flour
1 T. vanilla flavoring
Mix and spread over cereal mixture

Cake

2 c. spelt flour
1 c. fructose
1 t. soda
2 T. baking powder
1/2 t. cinnamon
1/2 t. allspice
1 egg
1/2 c. raisins
1/2 c. pecans or walnuts
3/4 c. cold water
1 1/2 c. shredded carrots

1 T. oil

Mix together and pour over mixture in bottom of pan. Bake 350° for 55-60 minutes or until toothpick comes out of the center clean.

RHUBARB DESSERT

3 c. fresh rhubarb
1 T. dry tapioca
28 drops stevia

Mix above ingredients and spread over bottom of 2-quart casserole dish.
1 c. oatmeal
1/2 c. 7 grain flour
1/3 c. fructose
1 egg

Mix until crumbly and spread over fruit mixture. Drop 1 1/2 T. butter over top of crumb mixture. Bake until fruit mixture bubbles up into crumb mixture, approximately 35-45 minutes.

PEACH CRISP

Mix and place into bottom of 9x9 inch pan:
6 peaches
1/4 c. honey
1/8 c. lemon juice
Sprinkle above with 1/4 t. cinnamon.
Mix together:
1 1/2 c. rolled oats
1/2 c. oat bran cereal

1/4 c. honey
1/2 c. butter
1/2 t. sea salt

Sprinkle over fruit mixture. Bake until fruit bubbles through the top mixture, approximately 35-45 minutes.

NUT TOSS

Mix together:
1 1/3 c. pecans
2 c. Almonds

In another bowl mix:
1 T. honey
1 T. sesame oil
1/4 t. cinnamon

Heat honey mixture in microwave on high 15-20 seconds. Stir and pour over nuts. Stir until all the nuts are coated. Spread nut mixture onto large brownie pan and bake 300° for 40-50 minutes. As nuts are cooling separate from bottom of pan with spatula 2-3 times to keep nuts from sticking to bottom of pan. Store in sealed container once nuts have cooled.

DELICIOUS NUT SNACK MIX

1/4 c. chopped dates
1/2 c. raisins
1/2 c. peanuts (unsalted)
1/2 c. pecan halves
1/2 c. sunflower seeds
1/2 c. filberts

1/2 c. cashews

Mix above ingredients and store in airtight container. If stored in the freezer it will keep for weeks.

FRENCH APPLE PIE

Pie Crust

3 c. buffalo flour
1/2 c. sunflower oil
1 c. water
3/4 t. sea salt

Mix flour, salt and oil with pastry cutter. Add water, a little at a time until dough is of pastry consistency. Roll 1/2 dough between 2 pieces of waxed paper. Place into pie tin.

Filling

Fill shell with slices of your favorite apple (pealed and sliced). Over apples dribble:

1 t. lemon juice
2 t. butter (melted with lemon juice)

Sprinkle over apples:
2-t. buffalo flour
3 T. cinnamon
1/8 c. fructose sugar

Roll out rest of pastry and place over fruit. seal edges by dipping finger into cold water and rubbing finger along top edge of pastry, then pinching top crust together with bottom crust. Make slits into top crust. Sprinkle 1 T. fructose over top of pie. Bake until apples bubble up through slits in crust, approximately 60-75 minutes.

APPLE PIE

Submitted by Pam Schramm

Place a large tortilla shell in the microwave for ten seconds and form the warm shell in the bottom of an eight-inch pie plate. Set aside. Peel, core, slice and cook 6 golden delicious or gala apples with:

3/4 c. water
1 c. raisins
3/4 c. pitted dates

Cook together on low until apples are cooked and water has evaporated.

Streusel Topping:
1/2 c. 7-grain bread crumbs
2 T. melted butter
1/2 t. cinnamon
1/8 t. nutmeg
1/8 t. allspice

Bake at 400° for 10 minutes. Turn oven down to 325° and bake for an additional 25-30 minutes. Let set, serve and enjoy.

HOLIDAY JEWELS

Submitted by Pam Schramm

1/2 c. unsweetened applesauce (made from gala apples)
1/3 c. raising

Combine and cover. Cook in microwave for 2 1/2 minutes on high. Stir after each minute. Prepare, cook and mash 1 c. squash or pumpkin. Add to above mixture and cook for two minutes in the microwave. Let cool.

Add:
1 egg white
1/2 t. vanilla

Mix together with cooled squash and raisin mixture. Then add the following dry ingredients to the above mixture:
1 1/4 c. 7 grain flour
1/2 c. unbleached white flour
1 t. soda
1 t. baking powder
1/2 t. flax seed
1/8 t. ginger
1/4 t. nutmeg
1/4 t. allspice
1/4 t. cinnamon

After mixing, drop by teaspoons onto cookie sheet. Make small indentation in center of each cookie and pace 1/2 t. of your favorite all-fruit jam. Enjoy the moist, cake-like cookie.

SUGAR-FREE OATMEAL COOKIES
Submitted by Yvonne Keeny

2 free-range eggs, beaten
2 c. unsweetened applesauce
1 t. powdered white stevia
1 t. nutmeg
1 t. cinnamon
2 t. baking soda
1 c. vegetable oil (not hydrogenated)
2 c. raisins
1 c. chopped nuts (walnuts are best)

2 1/2 c. oat flour
1 c. rolled oats
1 t. baking powder

Preheat oven to 325°. Stir together eggs, applesauce, stevia, nutmeg, cinnamon, baking soda and oil. Add raisins and nuts. Combine flour, oats and baking powder, then blend flour mixture into applesauce mixture. Drop by teaspoonfuls onto baking sheet. Bake 12 to 14 minutes or until golden brown. Makes about 5 dozen cookies.

OATMEAL DROP COOKIES

2 c. spelt flour
1 1/4 c. Fruitsource all purpose granular sweetener and fat replacer (Refer to "Sweeteners")
1 t. baking powder
1/2 t. soda
1 t. cinnamon
3 c. rolled oats
1 c. raisins
1 c. corn oil
2 eggs (beaten)
1/2 c. milk
3/4 t. stevia

Combine all dry ingredients and mix. Stir stevia into milk. To dry ingredients add remaining ingredients and mix. Bake in hot oven 400° for 10-12 minutes.

BANANA PUDDING

2 c. milk
3 T. cornstarch
3 eggs
1 T. water
1 t. vanilla
12 drops stevia
1 T. fructose
1 T. butter

Heat milk in a heavy saucepan. While milk is heating, separate eggs. To the yolks, add fructose, cornstarch and water. Slowly add yolk mixture to hot milk, stirring constantly. Bring up to a boil and boil just for a minute. Add vanilla and butter. Cool for 15 minutes. Add stevia. Cool and serve in a bowl over sliced bananas.

BANANA CAKE

2 c. oat flour
1/4 t. salt
1 c. mashed banana
2 t. baking powder
2 eggs
3 T. cold water
2 T. unrefined vegetable oil

Mix dry ingredients. Beat eggs. Add to the eggs the baking powder and cold water. Blend with dry ingredients and put batter into a greased 8x8-inch pan. Bake at 350° for 25-30 minutes.

ICE CREAM

(Although I don't suggest eating ice cream every day, I do indulge every few months. This ice cream is lower in sugar, and if it is made with skim milk, has a little less fat.)

2 eggs
2 c. skim milk (scalded)
1 t. vanilla
2 T. fructose
20 drops stevia
1/8 t. salt
1 1/2 c. evaporated milk, or half-and-half

Beat eggs until yolks and whites are well blended. Add fructose (not stevia) and salt, mixing well. Cook over medium low heat, stirring constantly until mixture begins to thicken. Chill. Add stevia, vanilla and evaporated milk or half-and-half. Freeze in ice cream freezer.

FRUIT CREAM (ice cream substitute)

2 oranges
2 c. fresh strawberries
1 c. plain, live culture yogurt
12 oz. frozen 100 percent cherry juice
Mix in blender. Freeze, stirring every 30 minutes. Eat in place of ice cream

FRUIT FREEZE (ice cream substitute)

2 oranges
2 bananas
2 nectarines

Blend in blender until smooth. Pour into a bowl and put into the freezer. Stir ever 2 hours until frozen.

FRUIT CRISP

Fill 1 1/2 quart casserole dish 3/4 full with fruit of your choice. Over fruit spread:
3/4 t. cinnamon
1/4 t. ground allspice

In a separate saucepan bring following ingredients to a boil until thickened:
2 T. cornstarch
1 c. apple, grape or cherry juice
1/4 c. fructose

After thickened, remove from heat and add:
10 drops stevia
Pour thickened mixture over the fruit. Top the fruit with the following mixture:
1 egg, beaten
2 T. butter, melted
1 c. rolled oats
1 c. kamut flakes
1/2 c. nuts of your choice
Bake at 350° for 45 minutes, or until fruit bubbles.

RHUBARB PHYLO ROLLS

In a sauce pan cook over low heat, 25 minutes or until fruit is softened:
1/2 c. water
1 lb. rhubarb
1 lb. strawberries
4 T. tapioca

Add:
2 T. corn starch mixed into 1/8 c. of water
Cook until fruit is thickened. Cool and add:
1 T. stevia

Separate 2 sheets phylo dough onto counter top or cookie sheet. Put 1/8 c. of fruit mixture onto the phylo dough and wrap dough up over fruit mixture. Place onto ungreased cookie sheet. Continue putting fruit mixture into dough and wrapping until all of fruit mixture is used. Bake roll ups for 20 minutes at 350°. Remove from oven and brush following mixture over the top of the roll ups:

3 T. butter (melted)
1/2 t. cinnamon
1/2 t. fructose

Return to the oven and bake another 10 minutes. Cool to set before serving.

EASY CARROT-SPICE CAKE

1 box fern spice cake mix
2 large carrots
Prepare box mix as directed using only 1/4 c. honey
instead of 1/2 c.

Frosting

4 oz. cream cheese, softened
1/4 c. butter, softened
1 1/2 T. honey
1/2 t. vanilla
Mix together and use for frosting.

RHUBARB GRAHAM DESSERT

Crust

8 graham crackers (crushed)
1/4 butter melted
1 T.. fructose
Mix together and press into a large pie shell. Bake at 350°
for 18 minutes. Meanwhile cook over medium heat:

4 cups fresh or frozen rhubarb
3/4 c. water
1/2 c. chopped nuts
1 T. oat flour
1/4 c. dark cherry concentrate or apple juice concentrate

Cook until thickened. Remove from heat and add 1 3/4
tsp. stevia. Stir into rhubarb mixture and pour into pie shell.
Cool.

Topping

1 c. heavy whipping cream
1/8 t. stevia
1/8 t. maple flavoring

Beat whipping cream, stevia, and maple flavoring until thick. Spread over rhubarb. Serve immediately. If you like vanilla flavoring, it may be substituted for maple flavoring.

EASY PIE CRUST

2 c. oat flour
1/4 t. sea salt
1/3 c. vegetable oil
2-3 T. Cold water

Roll out between 2 pieces of wax paper. Sprinkle little water under bottom piece to hold into place. This recipe makes 1 large pie crust, approximately 9 inch or better.

RICE AND RAISINS

1 c. rice
1 c. raisins
2 c. water
milk, about 3/4 c.
1 T. cinnamon
1 T. butter
stevia to sweeten

Place rice, raisins and water in medium saucepan. Cook, uncovered, over medium heat, stirring until liquid is almost gone. Remove from heat. Slowly add milk to cover rice, then cinnamon and butter. Stir together and add stevia to sweeten. Stir again and serve warm or chilled.

BAKED APPLES

4 large baking apples
1 c. nuts (walnuts or pecans)
1/2 t. cinnamon
1/4 t. allspice
Pinch nutmeg
1 t. vanilla
2 t. lemon juice
1 T. maple syrup
1/2 c. apple juice with 15 drops stevia

Heat oven to 350°. Wash and core apples. Cut 1/4 inch off bottom of cores to plug bottom of apple. Chop the nuts and mix together in a bowl with the maple syrup, vanilla and spices. Fill the apples with the mixture and pile it on the tops. Put the apples in a small baking dish. Mix the lemon juice, apple juice and stevia. Pour over the apples and cover the dish. Bake the apples until they are just beginning to soften—approximately 40 minutes. Do not overbake.

ALMOND DELIGHT

3/4 c. fresh coconut
3/4 c. almonds
1/2 c. unsweetened carob chips
1/8 t. stevia powder

Crack the shell of the coconut and drain off the juice. Peel the coconut from the shell and cut up into fine pieces. Add the almonds, carob and stevia. Stir until mixed up. Eat in a bowl with a spoon or freeze to eat as a snack.

CHEESECAKE

7-oz. pkg. amaranth graham crackers (crushed)
3/4 stick butter (melted)
12.3 oz. firm tofu
1/4 c. fat free sour cream
8 oz. fat free cream cheese
2 eggs
1 T. vanilla
2 T. fructose
21 drops stevia
1/4 c. Fruitsource Sweetener & Fat Replacer
2 1/2 c. fresh blueberries, fresh pineapple or fresh strawberries

Heat in the oven heat to 400°. Blend crackers and butter and press into cheesecake pan. Bake 350° for 10 minutes. Remove from oven and let set until cool. Mix tofu; sour cream, cream cheese, eggs, vanilla, fructose, stevia, and fruitsource. Blend until smooth. Fold in fruit and spread onto crust. Bake 400° 15 minutes. Lower oven temperature to 350° and bake another 55 minutes. Cool, to set up. This cheesecake is best when eaten 24 hours after baking.

VANILLA PUDDING

2-c. vanilla soy or rice milk
1 T. cornstarch
2 egg yolks
1/2 t. stevia
1 T. vanilla
1/2 t. salt

Beat egg yolks in a c.. Add 1/4 c. milk to egg yolks and mix together. Add cornstarch to egg mixture and blend.

Pour this mixture along with salt and remaining milk into a saucepan. Heat on low stirring constantly until bubbly and thick. Remove from heat and add the vanilla and stevia. Serve warm or cool.

BANANA PUDDING

2 bananas
Recipe of vanilla pudding

Make recipe of "Vanilla Pudding." Line the bottom of a bowl with bananas. Slice remaining bananas into pudding. Cool and serve.

Banana Cream Pie:

Place soft taco shell into pie tin. Poke with a fork and bake in 350° oven for 12 minutes or until slightly browned. Remove from oven and line bottom of shell with bananas. Pour pudding with remaining bananas into shell and return to the oven for another 20 minutes. Cool. Just before serving line top with another banana that has been sliced lengthwise.

PEACH ICE MILK

1 quart vanilla soy or rice milk
18 oz. firm tofu (1 1/2 cartons)
8 small ripe peaches
1/2 t. stevia or 1/2 T. fructose
1/2 can 100 percent apple/cherry concentrate

Blend milk and tofu in a blender. Pour into large bowl. Wash peaches and take the seed out. Put peaches and concentrates into the blender and blend until well blended. Add to the milk mixture and put into an ice cream freezer. Add rock salt and ice to freezer. Takes approximately 25 minutes to set. Makes approximately 8 servings.

NO BAKE CHEESECAKE

1 vanilla wafer "Keebler Ready Crust"
6 oz. fat free cream cheese
1/2 c. fat free sour cream
3/4 T. vanilla
12 drops stevia
4 oz. tofu
1 pint fresh fruit

Mix cream cheese, sour cream and tofu. Mix together vanilla and stevia. Add to the cheese mixture. Layer the bottom of the crust with fresh fruit. Pour cheese mixture over the fruit and layer with another layer of fruit. Chill for 2 hours to set.

Fruit Sauces and Toppings

Fruit sauces and toppings are wonderful for many uses. They work very nicely for toppings over pancakes and waffles. They are also delicious when dabbled over puddings, some pies and breads. Before reaching for syrup or honey, reach for fruit sauces and toppings. Your body will thank you!

RHUBARB SAUCE

2 quarts fresh rhubarb cut into 1/2 inch pieces
1/2 c. water
Boil without lid until rhubarb is tender and thickened.
Add:
1 T. liquid stevia
1 1/2 t. cinnamon

Cool and store in the refrigerator in a covered container.

STRAWBERRY SAUCE

2 quarts fresh strawberries
1/4 c. water

Boil until strawberries are tender and thickened. Add:
1/4 t. cinnamon
1/2 t. stevia
Mix and store in freezer or refrigerator.

APPLE SAUCE

2 quarts apples (pealed and cut into sections)
1/2 c. water
1 t. allspice

Boil over low heat until apples are tender. Remove from heat and mash. Add stevia drops until desired sweetness is achieved. Store in covered container in refrigerator of freezer.

CREAM CHEESE FROSTING

1/2 c. fat free cream cheese or rice cream cheese
1/3 c. Fruit Source Sweetener & Fat Replacer
1 1/2 T. butter, softened
1/4 t. cinnamon (optional)

Mix together and spread over cake.

APPLE DIP

6 oz. firm tofu
3/4 c. soy butter or peanut butter
1/8 t. powdered or 6 drops liquid stevia
1/2 t. vanilla

Blend in blender and use as apple dip. Delicious!

Drinks

APPLE SMOOTHIE DRINK

3 c. cold apple cider
2 T. wheat germ (Optional for those who are intolerant
    of wheat products)
2 bananas
1 small carton fat free, plain yogurt

Blend in blender and chill. Serve in chilled glasses.

RICH FRUIT SHAKE

1 small container plain yogurt
1/2 c. fruit juice of your choice
1 apple
1/2 c. frozen cherries
1/2 c. frozen peaches
2 T. flax seed

Blend in blender until smooth. Pour into glasses and top
with cherry or peach slice. Serves 2-3.

COOL QUENCHER

2 1/2 c. calcium-rich 100% orange juice
1 1/2 inch round slice from fresh pineapple
1 lb. bag whole, frozen strawberries

Blend together in blender. Serve with sprig of mint and cherry on top. Makes approximately 5 cups.

MINT TEA

This is a wonderful tea to help build the immune system as well as helping to soothe an upset stomach.
1/2 c. catnip leaves
1/2 c. mint leaves
2 quarts water

Heat water to boiling in the microwave. After water stops boiling, add the leaves. Let set for 15 minutes. Strain water through a strainer, or through a coffee strainer. Drink hot or add ice.

MINT TEA CUBES

Pick fresh mint and catnip leaves from garden. Wash carefully and place one of each leaf into ice cube squares in an ice cube tray. Fill tray with water and freeze. Use in fresh teas to cool for a summer treat.

APPLE MINT DRINK

2 mint tea bags
1 c. water (boiling)
1 quart 100 percent apple juice

Put tea bags into water and let set for 15 minutes. Add tea to apple juice. Chill and add Mint Tea Cubes. Place slice of apple over edge of jar.

STRAWBERRY PUNCH

1 can frozen orange/pineapple juice
1 can frozen strawberry juice
6 cans water

Mix and serve with ice ring in center of punch bowl.

ICE RING

1 bunt cake pan
sprigs of yarrow leaves
pansy flowers
sprigs of cilantro leaves (optional)

Fill cake pans about 1 inch deep with water. Pick leaves and flowers and set into pan, flower side down. Freeze. To remove from pan, tip pan upside down and run under hot water until ice ring falls out onto your hand.

HEALTH NUT TEA

1/4 c. mint leaves (chopped)
1/4 c. alfalfa leaves
1/4 c. catnip leaves (chopped)
1/4 c. lemon thyme leaves (chopped)

6 cups water that have been heated to boiling. Put leaves into the water and let set 10 to 15 minutes. Strain water and drink tea hot or cold.

FRUIT PUNCH

2 frozen container pineapple juice
1 frozen container apple juice
1 frozen container cherry juice

Mix juice in a gallon container. Add 12 cans of water. Chill and serve with an ice ring with orange slices frozen into the ice.

GINGER TEA

Ginger is a wonderful warming herb. It is said moderate amounts of ginger tea have the power to strengthen the lungs and kidneys.
6 c. water
1 1/2 inches ginger root
6 to 8 catnip tea bags
stevia

Bring water and ginger root to boil reducing heat. Simmer, covered for 5 minutes. Remove from heat. Add tea bags, let steep for 5 minutes. Remove tea bags. Strain ginger from tea. Add 3 to 5 drops stevia per cup of tea. Serve warm or over ice.

TOFU FRUIT SHAKE
Submitted by Anna Bell

3 oz. lowfat tofu
3/4 c. soy milk (vanilla)
1/2 c. fresh strawberries
1-4 drops stevia
7-8 ice cubes

Place all ingredients in blender and blend until smooth. Serve immediately. Can substitute blueberries, banana (add 1/4 t. nutmeg), peaches, apple or pineapple. Delicious.

APPLE SMOOTHIE DRINK

3 c. cold apple cider
2 T. wheat germ (optional for those who are intolerant of wheat products)
2 bananas
1 small carton fat free, plain yogurt

Blend in blender and chill. Serve in chilled glasses.

EASY BREAKFAST DRINK

1/2 c. favorite 100 percent fruit juice
2 T. oatmeal
1 T. wheat germ
1 1/2 T.. Flax seed
1 Banana
3 other fresh fruits of your choice (peaches, oranges, pears, etc.)

Blend together in blender until creamy. Top with cherry. Serves 2.

RICH FRUIT SHAKE

1 small container plain yogurt
1/2 c. fruit juice of your choice
1 apple
1/2 c. frozen cherries

1/2 c. frozen peaches
2 T. flax seed

Blend in blender until smooth. Pour into glasses and top
with cherry or peach slice. Serves 2-3.

Main Dishes
and Soups

ITALIAN CASSEROLE

One 10 1/2-oz. Jar MSG free Spaghetti Sauce
4 med.-lrg. potatoes
1 medium onion
2 cloves garlic
1 1/2 lb. ground turkey
2 qt. Casserole dish with cover

Pour 1/2 c. spaghetti sauce over bottom of casserole dish.
Layer ingredients in this manner: meat, onions, garlic, potatoes, sauce, meat, onions, potatoes, sauce. Finish with layer
of sauce. Bake 400° for 90 minutes. (A double batch of this
casserole can be made and baked and put into the freezer to
be heated for a later meal.)

"FISHLESS" FILLETS

Freeze 1 pkg. tofu, thaw, and squeeze out excess water
with a paper towel. Cut into 6 equal slices.

1 c. bread or cracker crumbs
1 T. parmesan cheese
1/4 t. garlic salt
1/4 t. onion powder
1/4 t. paprika

Baste fillets with olive oil. Roll in mix and bake for 20
minutes at 350°. Serve in a bun as a fish fillet.

DELICIOUS BURRITOS

1 can refried beans
1 pkg. taco seasoning (MSG-free)
1/2 c. picante sauce
Mix above ingredients over medium heat until warm.

1 package fat free cheddar cheese
One 10 oz. container fat free sour cream
1 med. tomato
1 small onion
1 sm. Can ripe olives
3/4 c. shredded lettuce
3/4 c. shredded spinach
3 T. picante sauce

Meanwhile warm taco shells in microwave on high for 15 seconds. Bring shells out of microwave and add beans. Before folding shell over beans, add on top of beans equal portions of the rest of the toppings listed above. Fold taco shell. Turn shells upside down on plate so fold is under shell. On top of each shell put 1 T. sour cream and a couple pieces of the chopped tomato. Sprinkle with 1 t. cheddar cheese.

SWEET AND SPICY CHICKEN

2 c. diced cooked chicken
2 T. oil
1 turnip (peeled and diced)
1 apple (diced)
5 medium mushrooms (diced)
sauté above ingredients for 10 minutes.

Add:
2 c. chunky medium salsa
8 oz tomato sauce (no salt added)
2 T. brown rice malt syrup
1/2 t. salt

Add remaining ingredients and simmer 25 minutes. Serve over steamed rice or cooked barley. Serves 4-5.

TEXAS TATER WEDGES

14 low fat Ritz crackers
3 T. humus dip (can be found in health food stores)

Mix together and pour into a pie pan.
3 T. olive oil (put into a bowl)
5 medium potatoes

Wash potatoes in Shaklee Basic H to remove chemicals. Scrub and cut into wedges. Roll in olive oil and then in cracker mixture. Bake at 350° for 35-40 minutes or until tender. Serves 5

MEAT LOAF PIE

1 lb. ground beef
2 c. reconstituted vegetable protein
3/4 c. oats
1 egg, beaten
1/4 c. chopped onion
2 cloves chopped garlic
1/3 c. water
1 t. salt
1/2 t. pepper

Combine ingredients. Push into 8x8-inch baking dish or 2 quart casserole dish, leaving a hollow area in the middle of the meat. Into the hollow dice the following vegetables:

2 potatoes, peeled
2 carrots
1/2 c. corneal corn
Bake 350° for about 1 hour.
Double the recipe, bake and freeze for another meal. Serves 6.

MEAT LOAF

1 c. ground chuck
2 T.. worcestershire sauce
1 c. TVP (Texturized Vegetable Protein) hydrated
1/4 c. onion, minced
1/4 t. cumin
1/2 c. catsup
1/4 c. crackers
1/2 c. oatmeal
2 T. mustard

Mix above ingredients. Shape into loaf and put into a 2-quart casserole dish. Cover with "topping" and bake 350° until done.

Topping

1/4 c. catsup
3 T. sucunot sugar

GRILLED SALMON

2 lb. salmon steaks
3/4 c. butter, melted
1/4 c. lemon juice
1/4 c. fresh cilantro leaves
Hot charcoals for grilling.

Place frozen salmon steaks on aluminum foil on top of grill with hot charcoals. Mix butter and lemon juice and minced cilantro leaves. Baste steaks with butter mixture. Place cover on grill. Turn steaks after 10 minutes. Pour 1 T. butter over each steak. Continue basting steaks with butter until steaks are tender, approximately 20-25 minutes.

EASY COD FILETS

Heat oven to 350°. Place 10 pieces frozen cod into baking dish or pan. Bake 25 minutes. Take out of the oven and top with:

1 c. fat free mayonnaise
1/2 c. low fat Ritz crackers (crushed)

Squeeze 1 fresh lemon over fish and topping. Bake an additional 15 minutes or until fish is tender and flaky.

CABBAGE AND MEAT BALLS

1 medium head cabbage, washed and shredded
1/2 lb. ground chuck
1 c. uncooked wild rice
1 c. reconstituted TVP (Texturized Vegetable Protein)
salt and pepper to taste

Wash and shred cabbage. Place in heavy kettle. In a bowl combine ground beef, TVP, rice, salt and pepper. Make walnut-sized meat balls, and add to pot. Add water to cover, and place lid on pot. Simmer over medium heat until meatballs are cooked through and rice is tender, 30-40 minutes. Do not stir, or meatballs will fall apart.

RICE DINNER

2 c. cooked long grain rice
1 medium onion
1 sm. clove garlic
2 T. butter
1 bunch broccoli (cut into pieces)
1/2 c. blanched almonds
1/2 c. fat free Parmesan cheese

Sauté onion and garlic in butter. Stir in remaining ingredients except cheese. Heat until mixture is hot. Sprinkle with cheese and serve.

MEATLESS MEAT LOAF

4 c. reconstituted TVP
1/2 c. worcestershire sauce
3 T. beef bouillon
3 1/2 c. water

Bring to a boil and add:
1/2 medium onion
1 med. garlic clove
3/4 c. catsup
3 T. mustard
3/4 can MSG free cream of mushroom soup
1/2 c. gluten flour

Mix above ingredients together and pat into 2-quart glass casserole dish.

Topping

1/2 c. catsup
2 T. mustard
1/2 t. stevia

Spread over meat loaf and bake 350° for approximately 1 hour 20 minutes.

VEGETARIAN PIZZA

Crust

1/3 c. oat flour
1/3 c. brown rice flour
1/3 c. gluten free flour
2 t. baking powder
1/3 c. flax seed meal
1/4 t. sea salt
1/3-c. soy or rice milk
1 egg

Mix together above ingredients except gluten free flour. Add enough gluten flour to make a soft dough consistency. Press dough onto a greased pizza pan sprinkling gluten flour lightly on top of dough to keep it from sticking onto your fingers.

Topping for dough

Brush 1 T. olive oil over dough. Add:
Green peppers; garlic (1 clove); onion; whole, ripe tomatoes; ripe olives; 1/2 t. thyme; 2 basil leaves chopped. Bake

375° for 15 minutes. Take out of the oven and top with 1 package fat free pizza cheese. Return to the oven and bake another 15 minutes.

SPIRAL VEGGIE DINNER

8 oz. kamut spirals
Boil 7 to 10 minutes or until tender. Set aside.
2 T. olive oil
2 medium garlic cloves
1 small onion

Brown garlic and onion in oil. Add:
2 carrots, diced
1 celery stick, diced
1 c. broccoli (fresh)
1/2 c. fresh parsley
1/4 c. fresh chives
1 c. cauliflower
1/8 c. parmesan cheese

Stir vegetables into onion and garlic over medium heat, stirring constant until crisp-tender. Toss. (Optional: Top dinner with spaghetti or cheese sauce.

SOUTHWESTERN BEANS AND RICE

2 c. cold cooked long grain rice
1 can kidney beans, rinsed and drained
1 can (8 1/2 oz.) whole kernel corn, drained
1/2 c. chopped onion
1/2 c. picante sauce
3/4 c. salad oil

3/4 c. catsup
1/2 c. vinegar
1/4 t. powder stevia

Cook the rice and rinse. Combine rice, beans corn onion and picante sauce. Stir. In another bowl combine salad oil, catsup, vinegar, and stevia. Whip together until well blended. Pour over rice mixture. Serve warm or cold.

MEXICAN CHIPS

(This is a great meal to enjoy a couple of times per month. Because has some foods that are more highly processed we usually have it on special occasions when we feel like "splurging".)

1 bag fat free tortilla chips
1 lb. tofu cheddar cheese
1 can black olives (chopped)
1 can refried beans (you can make your own)
2 tomatoes
1/2 medium onion, chopped
2-4 fresh jalapeño peppers
fat free sour cream

Pour half of the chips onto a large cookie sheet. Spread 1/2 of the beans on top. Over beans sprinkle half of the rest of the ingredients except sour cream. Place into a 350° oven for 5 minutes. Take out of the oven and top with remaining ingredients except sour cream. Return to the oven for another 15 minutes or until cheese is melted. Top with sour cream and serve with tofu shake for a great summer meal.

LASAGNA

1 box brown rice lasagna noodles

Cook noodles into boiling water 7 to 10 minutes or until done. Mix together:
1 small container ricotta cheese
1 egg
1/2 t. sea salt
1/4 t. pepper

Set aside. Mix these ingredients together in a separate bowl:
2 cloves garlic
1 medium onion
1 lb. fresh spinach
1 tomato
1 bell pepper
1 red pepper
1 jar spaghetti sauce with thyme

Spread 2 T. spaghetti sauce onto bottom of 9x13-inch pan. Layer noodles over sauce. Add 1/4 of remaining spaghetti sauce. Spread 1/2 of ricotta sauce over spaghetti sauce, then 1/2 of vegetables. Finish layering ingredients, ending with sauce over top of the top layer of noodles. Cover with 1 package of fat free mozzarella cheese. Bake 350° approximately 40-45 minutes, or until sauce bubbles.

BBQ TURNOVERS

1 1/2 c. water
2 small cloves garlic
1 medium onion

1/2 t. sea salt

Bring above ingredients to a boil. Turn off heat and add:
1 1/2 c. TVP

Let above mixture set, stirring occasionally while mixing together next ingredients:
2 c. whole oat flour
1 c. gluten free flour
1/2 t. sea salt
2 t. baking powder
1/2 c. sunflower oil

Mix dry ingredients. Cut in oil. Add cold water, 1 T. at a time until dough forms a soft, moist, ball. Set aside. To TVP add:
1/4 c. brown sugar
3/4 c. catsup
3 t. worcestershire sauce

Separate dough into 8 balls. Roll each ball between waxed paper like a piecrust. Place tomato slice on one side of the dough. Add 1/4 to 1/3 c. TVP mixture over tomato. Fold over other half and seal edges. With a fork, poke holes into the top of the crust. Bake 400° until juice bubbles out of the holes.

MEXICAN CHICKEN AND RICE

1 lb. chicken breast
1 T. olive oil
1/3 c. onions
1/2 c. green peppers
1 clove garlic

14-1/2 oz stewed tomatoes
1/2 c. green chilies
14 1/2 oz fat free chicken broth
2 c. brown rice
1/4 t. hot sauce
1 1/2 T. non-fat plain yogurt
1 c. celery
1/2 c. red sweet peppers
7 T. black olives

Dice celery, onions, green peppers, green chilies and clove of garlic. Cook rice in hot water for about 15 minutes. In large skillet cook chicken in olive oil about 3 minutes on each side until brown. Remove and set aside in the same skillet, cook onion, peppers and garlic until tender but not brown. Drain off fat. Stir in undrained tomatoes, broth, rice, celery, and hot sauce. Bring to boiling; remove from heat and spoon mixture into a 1 by 7 1/2 by 2 inch baking dish. Arrange chicken on top of rice mixture. Bake covered, in 350° oven for 30 to 35 minutes or until rice is done. Sprinkle with olives; top with yogurt. Serves 6.

HOLIDAY CHICKEN

5 large chicken breasts
1/2 T. mustard   .
1 t. cilantro leaves
1 sm. clove garlic
1/2 c. apple juice
1/8 t. ground nutmeg

Mix all ingredients but chicken breasts. Place chicken breasts into container with sealing lid. Pour liquid mix over chicken and gently turn container until all chicken pieces are coated. Let set 3 hours in refrigerator, turning every hour. Place chicken into a casserole dish and pour sauce and spices over the top of chicken. Bake 350° for 45 minutes or until done.

CORNBREAD CHILE

1-15 oz. can of organic chili
1-15 oz. can pork and beans
1 T. chili powder
1 c. cornmeal
1 cup oat flour
1 T. honey
1 t. salt
1/8 cup flaxseed, ground
3/4 t. baking soda
1 t. baking powder
2 eggs, well beaten
1/4 c. vegetable oil
1 1/2 c. rice or soy milk

Combine chile, beans and chile Powder in 2-quart casserole dish. Mix the remaining ingredients and pour over bean mixture. Bake 350° for 45 minutes or until corn bread mixture is lightly brown and done.

BBQ CASSEROLE

2 c. water
2 cloves garlic
1/2 med. onion

Bring above ingredients to a boil and add:
1/2 green pepper

3 T. worcestershire sauce
3/4 c. catsup
2-t. chili powder.
1/2 T. sucanot sugar
2 T. mustard
2 c. TVP

Let set 10 minutes. Add:
1 can baked beans
Set aside.

Crust

1 c. whole wheat flour
1 c. oat flour
1/2 c. wheat germ
2 T. flax meal
2 T. baking powder.

Mix above ingredients together. Cut in:
1/4 c. olive oil
1/2 t. sea salt

Add:
1/2 c. water

Mix in water until flour mixture is moistened. Divide dough in half. Press half of dough into bottom of 2-quart casserole dish. Add vegetable mixture. Roll out remaining dough to form to casserole dish. Place on top of vegetables. Bake 350° until vegetable mixture bubbles.

DINNER CASSEROLE

1 c. cornmeal flour
1/4 c. flax meal
3/4 c. 10 grain flour
1 T. baking powder
1 egg, beaten
1/2 t. soda
1 c. water
8 drops stevia
1/2 t. sea salt
3/4 c. frozen corn

Mix water and stevia. Add remaining of above ingredients. Stir together and set aside.

Sauté in hot skillet:
1 T. oil
2 red peppers (diced)
1 onion (diced)
2 cloves garlic

Heat to boiling:
2 1/4 c. water
2 T. worcestershire sauce
2 T. maple syrup
1 t. mustard

Remove from heat and add:
2 c. TVP
1/2 c. catsup
2 T. vinegar

Add vegetables and stir together with TVP mixture. Pour into 2-quart casserole dish. Pour cornbread mixture over top. Bake uncovered 400° until cornbread mixture is done.

MEXICAN PIZZA

Crust:
1/4 c. barley malt flour
1/2 c. flaxseed flour
1 1/4 c. oat flour
1/4 c. spelt flour
2 t. baking powder.
2 T. sunflower oil
1 egg, beaten
1/2 t. sea salt
1/4 c. water

Mix together and let set 3-5 minutes. Press onto a lightly greased round pizza pan.
1 garlic clove
3 tomatoes
1 medium onion
1 hot pepper
1 can refried beans1
pkg. fat free pizza cheese

Mince vegetables. Sprinkle onto crust. Bake 10 minutes in a 400° oven. Reduce heat to 350° and bake another 25 minutes. Remove pizza from oven and add cheese. Return to the oven and bake another 10 minutes.

BREAKFAST PIZZA

Prepare crust as for Mexican pizza. Bake 350° for 10 minutes. When crust comes out of the oven, layer cheddar cheese on top of crust.

1 T. olive oil
1/2 t. salt
1/2 c. onions
1/2 c. green pepper
1 clove garlic
1 t. sage
1/2 t. parsley
8 eggs
1 t. sage
8 slices fat free cheddar
1 c. tofu mozzarella cheese
cheese

Sauté vegetables and spices in oil. In a separate bowl beat eggs until yolks and whites are blended. Pour over vegetables and cook over medium heat, stirring constantly until moist, but cooked. Spread over crust and cheese. Top with mozzarella cheese and bake 350° 10 minutes or until cheese is melted.

QUICK, EASY EGG TORTILLAS

6 eggs from range chickens
1 clove garlic
1/4 c. chopped onion
1/4 c. chopped pepper
salt and pepper to taste
5 tortilla shells

Sauté garlic, onion and green pepper in 1 T. olive oil until slightly crisps (about 2 minutes). Add eggs, salt and pepper and scramble until eggs are cooked. Divide and wrap into tortilla shells, adding your favorite picante sauce. If you would like to save these for another meal, omit picante sauce, wrap in plastic wrap and freeze. To eat, microwave until heated through and add picante sauce.

BREAKFAST "McMUFFINS"

4 eggs (range)
4 slices fat free Swiss cheese
4 whole wheat English muffins
1 T. olive oil

Fry eggs in oil. Separate each muffin and place one piece of cheese on each muffin. Set fried egg on cheese and add the top of the muffin. These can be wrapped in plastic wrap and frozen for later meals. Thaw and heat in microwave.

RICE-N-SPINACH SALAD

1 1/2 c. cooked long grained rice
2 heads broccoli (cut into pieces)
1 lb. fresh spinach (chopped into pieces)
1 small garlic clove

Steam broccoli until crisp tender. Rinse with cool water until cool. Combine above ingredients.

Dressing

1 c. oil
10 drops stevia

1/3 c. ketchup
2 T. worcestershire sauce
1/4 c. chopped onion

Mix all ingredients in dressing using a wire wisk. (Will take awhile to get all ingredients mixed.) Pour over salad, stirring to cover all ingredients. Serve warm or chilled.

EASY ONE-DISH MEAL

1 organically grown roast (whatever size you need)
5 carrots, peeled
4 large potatoes, peeled
1 large onion
1 medium garlic, minced
1 stalk of celery
1 c. water
1 1/2 t. salt
1/2 t. pepper
2 T. lemon thyme

Pour water into a pan large enough to hold all of the above ingredients. Add roast, salt, pepper, and half of onion, garlic ad thyme. Layer remaining ingredients on top of roast. Bake 350° for 4 hours.

LAMB STEW

3/4 lb. fresh lamb pieces
1 med. onion

Brown lamb and onion in 2 T. olive oil. Rinse meat with hot water to remove grease and oils. Put into 2-quart crock-pot and add:

2 c. water
1 1/2 t. rosemary sprigs

Cook in crock pot 12 hours or until meat is very tender. Rinse and drain meat. Add as much water to meat as you want. Add diced vegetables to fill pot:

potatoes
carrots
garlic (2 cloves)
onion (one)
peas
1/2 c. chic peas

Cook in slow cooker 12 hours. salt and pepper to taste.

VEGETABLE BEAN SOUP

6 potatoes, peeled and diced
1 onion, chopped
3 celery stalks, chopped
6 c. water
2 MSG free beef bouillon cubes
1 c. pinto beans
1 c. whole corn
1 c. green beans
1 c. carrots, diced
1 can pork and beans
1 (10.5-ounce) can tomatoes
1 c. peas
2 c. cabbage, shredded (optional)
1 onion
1 clove garlic

Combine potatoes, celery, onion, water and bouillon cubes in pot over high heat. Cook until vegetables are tender. Add salt to taste. Add rest of vegetables, soup and if desired cabbage. Heat through and serve. (Freezes well.) Makes approximately 24 servings.

VEGETABLE SOUP

Soak in hot water 60 minutes:
3/4 c. red beans
3/4 c. pinto beans
Boil 60 minutes, drain and add:
1 lb. organically grown beef stew chunks
4 c. water
1 onion
1 clove garlic
2 potatoes, peeled
2 carrots, peeled
salt and pepper to taste

Cook in a crock-pot over night or 12 hours. Serve with baking powder biscuits.

TURKEY/CELERY SOUP

1 1/2 quarts water
2 c. organically grown left over turkey pieces (from roasted or baked turkey)
4 celery sticks and leaves, cleaned and minced
5 medium carrots, cleaned and diced
2 T. dried parsley (1 T. fresh parsley)
1 mint tea bag
1 T. butter
juice from 1/4 lemon

1/2 c. wild rice
salt and pepper to taste

Combine above ingredients and simmer 2 hours. Remove
tea bag and serve hot.

BEAN SOUP

1 c. pinto beans
1 c. calico lima beans
1 c. red kidney beans

Soak beans I hot water 1 hour. Drain and add:
2 large cloves garlic
1 medium onion
3 tomatoes, peeled
2 large carrots, cleaned and diced
1 celery stalk, cleaned and diced
10 broccoli spears, cleaned and cut into pieces
1/4 c. fresh parsley
3 T. fresh sage
3 t. sea salt
1/4 t. pepper
2 c. water

Simmer above ingredients on low heat for 2-3 hours, or
until beans are soft and cooked.

FRENCH ONION SOUP

5 lbs. yellow onions thinly sliced
6 T. butter
2 T. olive oil
1/2 t. sugar

2 t. salt
1/4 c. + 1 T. flour
14 c. boiling beef broth
1 1/2 c. dry white wine
whole grain bread to soak
fat-free Swiss and parmesan cheese

Simmer onions in butter and olive oil in stockpot for 2
hours, stirring frequently. Add sugar and salt after 15 minutes of cooking. Onions will be golden brown. Sprinkle
flour on onions and cook 5 minutes. Add boiling broth and
wine and simmer another 45 minutes, skimming top if necessary. Ladle into bowls and add cheese over top of each
bowl. Serve with bread. Makes about 16 cups.

CABBAGE ROLLS

1 c. barley (cooked)
1 c. basmati or jasmine rice (cooked)
1 can sauerkraut (drained)
1 c. spaghetti sauce
1 garlic clove, minced
1/4 c. chopped onion
1 head of cabbage

Mix first six ingredients. Gently peel off leaves of cabbage. Fill leaves with barley mixture and roll. Place into
cake pan with 1/4 c. water in the bottom. Bake 1 hour at
350°.

Salads

CARROT SALAD

2 c. shredded carrots
1/8 c. crushed pineapple
1/8 c. raisins
2 T. fat free cholesterol free mayonnaise

Mix and refrigerate 2 hours before serving. Is fresh for up to 3 days when refrigerated.

DINNER SALAD

2 c. vegetable pasta (cooked)
1 carrot, cleaned and minced
1 celery stick, cleaned and minced
1/4 c. green pepper
1 clove garlic, minced
1 t. lemon thyme
3/4 c. peas
3/4 c. fat free, Canola Mayo
1/2 c. water
9 drops stevia

Mix vegetables and pasta together in a bowl. Combine thyme, garlic, mayonnaise, water and stevia. Pour over vegetables and pasta. Chill.

CABBAGE SLAW (sour)

1/2 head cabbage
1/2 t. mustard seed
3/4 c. vinegar
2 t. dill seed
3/4 c. dill relish
1/4 c. Bread-n-Butter pickle juice

Shred cabbage into a bowl. Mix remaining ingredients and pour over the cabbage. Store in refrigerator up to 3 days.

CABBAGE/CARROT SLAW

1/2 head cabbage
4 carrots (cleaned)
1 stick celery

Shred above ingredients in a food processor and pour into a bowl. Refrigerate until ready to use.

To make salad to eat:

Dish salad out into a bowl. To each bowl of salad, add 1 1/2 T. of your favorite slaw dressing. If you would like to sweeten the slaw dressing, add 5-10 drops stevia to dressing before pouring over the salad.

HEALTH SALAD

1 1/2 C. frozen peas
1/2 c. frozen corn
3/4 c. brown rice (cooked)

1 c. short grain rice (cooked)
4 eggs (hard boiled and peeled)

Dressing
2 Tbsp sweet pickle relish
1/4 C. fat free thousand island dressing
(serves 4-5)
Combine vegetables, rice, and eggs. Cover with dressing.
Serve at room temperature or chilled.

CUCUMBER SALAD

4 cucumbers (7-8 inches long)
6 T. red wine vinegar
1/4 c. raw shallots, chopped
1 sm. Clove garlic
2 T. chopped chives
2 T. water
1/4 t. Black pepper
3 1/2 T. dill weed
5 drops stevia

Peel cucumbers and finely shred. Place strands in a colander; sprinkle with 1 tablespoon vinegar. Let stand 40 minutes. Shake colander to remove excess liquid. Put into bowl
and add shallots, clove and chives. Combine remaining
vinegar, stevia, 2 tablespoons dill and water. Mix and pour
over vegetables. Toss lightly with 2 forks. Cover and refrigerate 15-30 minutes. Sprinkle with remaining dill.

CHEFS SALAD

(Serves 2)
2 c. shredded leaf lettuce
2 c. shredded spinach leaves
2 large carrots, cleaned and shredded
1/2 c. shredded cucumber
1/2 c. green pepper
1/2 c. shredded zucchini squash
1/4 c. shredded parsley
1-stalk celery including leaf tops (cut into small pieces)
1/4 c. red bell pepper
2 hard boiled eggs
2 T. unsalted sesame seeds
2 T. sunflower seeds
2 T. favorite dressing

Combine all ingredients except eggs and seeds. Pour dressing on top of salad. Slice eggs and place on top of salad. Sprinkle with seeds.

4 BEAN SALAD

1/2 c. pinto beans (dry)
1/2 c. garbanzo beans (dry)
1/2 c. baby lima beans

Soak beans in warm water for 1 hour. Drain, rinse and cover with water. Bring to a boil and simmer until beans are soft, approximately 1-hour. Drain and add:

1 c. frozen green beans
1/2 c. chopped onion
1 small clove garlic (optional)

Combine all of the above ingredients and mix well.

Dressing

1/2 c. red wine salad vinegar
1/4 c. salad oil
1 t. stevia
1/4 t. pepper
1/4 t. lemon juice

Mix ingredients for dressing well. Pour over the beans and store in an airtight container. Tip the container upside down a number of times to cover the beans with dressing. Cool for at least 2 hours before serving.

FRUIT PALETTE

2 medium apples
2 bananas
1 c. blackberries

Mix together and set aside. Meanwhile put remaining ingredients into a saucepan and heat until thickened:
3/4 c. apple cider
1/4 c. orange juice
2 T. corn starch

Pour over the fruit mixture. Serve warm or chilled.

BASIC FRUIT SALAD

1 apple
1 banana
1 c. sweet cherries
1 peach

1 T. lemon juice
1/4 c. water
15 drops stevia

Cut above fruits into a bowl. Mix lemon juice, water and stevia. Pour over fruit and serve. (More or less stevia can be added to taste.)

FRUIT DESSERT SALAD

1 pint basket strawberries
3 kiwi fruit
1 medium cantaloupe
1 medium honey dew melon
1/4 c. mint leaves (chopped)
1/4 c. pecans
1/2 c. fresh orange juice
1/4 c. fresh lemon juice
10 drops stevia

Wash, drain and hull strawberries. Peel kiwis and slice thin, reserving 1 sliced kiwi for garnish. Slice melons into small squares, or cut with melon baller. Mix all fruits together except for reserved kiwi. Chop mint leaves and tender stems very fine and sprinkle on fruits. Mix orange and lemon juice with stevia and pour over all. Sprinkle with nuts. Arrange reserved kiwi slices on top and garnish with fresh mint. Chill 2-3 hours and serve cold.

CUCUMBER SALAD

1 medium cucumber
1 medium onion
1/2 c. oil

3 T. lemon juice
2 T. dill leaves

Peel and slice cucumber and onion into a bowl. Mix oil,
lemon juice and dill. Pour over vegetables. Put into the
refrigerator to marinate vegetables for at least 2 hours
before serving.

PARTY FRUIT SALAD

1/2 c. frozen orange juice concentrate
1 banana
1 pkg. frozen mixed fruit

Blend orange juice concentrate and banana. Pour as
dressing over fruit. Thaw and serve.

BROCCOLI SALAD

3 c. broccoli tops
1-c. carrots (cut in pieces)
1 celery stick, minced
1 green pepper, chopped
3 hard boiled eggs, chopped
2 T. onion (chopped)
3/4 c. fat free mayonnaise
2 T. Balsamic vinegar
1/4 c. water

Steam broccoli and carrots until crisp tender. Drain and
rinse in cool water. Mix mayonnaise vinegar and water until
well blended. Pour over vegetables and mix well. Chill
before serving.

THREE BEAN SALAD

1 can pinto beans
1 can red beans
1 can green beans
1 garlic clove (minced)
1 small onion (minced)
1/2 c. balsamic vinegar
1/4 c. canola oil
15 drops stevia

Stir vegetables together. Mix oil, stevia, and vinegar until well mixed. Pour over vegetables and chill.

Dressings

THICK RICH MAYONNAISE

(For egg salads tuna or fish)
4 large garlic cloves
1/4 c. eggs (approximately 1 egg)
1-2 T. lemon juice
1/4 t. salt
3/4 c. olive or salad oil

In blender combine garlic, egg lemon juice and salt. Process 5 seconds; gradually add oil in thin steady stream. Pour mixture into covered container and refrigerate up to 3 days. Can add green onion or dill to change flavor.

CHIP DIP

8 oz. piquant sauce
8 oz. Organic refried beans

Mix together and use for baked potato or corn chips.

THOUSAND ISLAND DRESSING

3/4 c. fat free, MSG free mayonnaise
1/4 c. catsup
2 T. sweet pickle relish

Mix together and store in covered container in refrigerator. Will keep up to one week.

HONEY MUSTARD DRESSING

1/2 c. fat free, MSG free mayonnaise
1 t. mustard
3/4 c. water
5 drops Steve

Mix together until smooth. Mixture will thicken. Store in refrigerator. (Makes approximately 3/4 c.)

MINNY SKINNY DIP

Vegetables of your choice for dipping.
1/4 t. mustard
1 t. minced onion
1/8 t. minced garlic
1/2 t. water
8 oz. Lowfat plain yogurt
1/2 t. paprika
1/2 t. dill weed

Combine mustard, onion, garlic and water; set aside for a few minutes to develop flavor. Mix together the rest of the ingredients. Stir in onion and mustard mixture. Chill until ready to serve.

EASY DOES IT SOUR CREAM

2 T. skim milk
1 T. lemon juice
1 c. lowfat cottage cheese

Mix above ingredients in the blender until smooth and creamy.

MAYONNAISE

1/2 c. eggs (approximately 2 small or
1 large)
1/2 t. mustard
1/2 t. sugar
1/4 t. paprika
2 T. white vinegar
1 c. oil
Combine eggs, mustard, sugar, paprika, vinegar and 1/2 c. oil in blender. Blend, just until mixed. While blender continues to blend the ingredients, pour in remaining ingredients in a slow, steady stream. Use spatula to keep mixture flowing. Blend until mixture is completely blended and smooth. Store in the refrigerator.

SWEET-N-SOUR SALAD

(Fresh cooked beans can be substituted
for the canned beans.)
1 can black eyed peas
1 can red beans
1 can northern beans
1 can sauerkraut
1/2 medium onion, minced
3/4 t. chili pepper
1/2 t. stevia
Mix beans and onion together in a bowl. Drain juice from sauerkraut into a cup. To sauerkraut juice add chili pepper and stevia. Mix and pour over the bean mixture. Refrigerate at least 2 hours before serving.

Vegetables

HERBED VEGETABLES

(4 servings)
Steam for 18 minutes:
4 long carrots (cleaned & cut into 1 inch pieces
3 potatoes (peeled)

Meanwhile sauté in 2 T. butter:
1 medium onion
1 lrg. Garlic clove

Add potatoes & carrots to onion mixture.
Mix together:
1 t. Rosemary
1/2 t. Basil
Toss onto potato mixture, serve hot.

DELICIOUS GRILL

1 onion (cut into large pieces)
4 carrots (cut into 1-inch diagonal pieces)
1/4 head cabbage (cut into large pieces)
3 broccoli tops cut up
2 medium size garlic cloves
1/2 c. fresh parsley
1/2 c. fresh lemon thyme (minced)
2 TBSP. olive oil
Charcoals on grill
heavy iron skillet

Place iron skillet on coals with oil in it. As soon as skillet is hot put vegetables into it. Put the cover over the grill and let vegetables cook, stirring occasionally to keep from burning. Serve hot.

BAKED POTATOES

To create a wonderful, yet easy meal, begin with 4 large potatoes that have been scrubbed. Put them into a casserole dish with 3 T. water. Cover and bake in a 400-degree oven for approximately 1 hour or until soft. Serve the potatoes topped with any of the following toppings:

Barbecue TVP (one of our favorites)
Picante Sauce and Plain yogurt
Spaghetti Sauce
onions and garlic sautéed in butter and topped with spaghetti sauce.
Tuna Salad
Broccoli and fat free cheese
Pork and Beans
Beans of any kind

Experiment on your own. There are no rights or wrongs in cooking, only "new" experiences. Enjoy this new adventure, it is a lot of fun!

BAKED SWEET POTATOES

4 large sweet potatoes
Mix together:
1/2 c. butter, softened
1 t. cinnamon
1/2 t. stevia

Bake potatoes with skins on, in casserole bowl with 4 T. water. When tender, take potatoes out of the oven and cut in half. Mash through the center of the potato and top with butter topping.

STUFFED POTATOES

6 large potatoes
1/2 c. butter (soft)
8 oz. Fat free sour cream
2 oz. Fat free cream cheese (softened)
1 c. fat free grated cheddar cheese
1 t. salt
1/4 t. pepper
paprika

Bake potatoes; remove from shell and ad rest of ingredients. Sprinkle with paprika. Return to oven for 7 minutes.

GREEN BEAN CASSEROLE

1 bag frozen green beans
1/2 c. chopped onion
1/2 t. salt
1/4 t. pepper
1 can MSG free cream of mushroom soup

Mix above ingredients in a casserole dish. Bake at 350° until bubbly.

TEXAS TOMATOES

4 potatoes, peeled and cut into wedges
1-c. saltine cracker crumbs
1/2 t. garlic powder
1/2 t. paprika
1/2 t. onion powder.
3 T. olive oil

Mix crackers, garlic, paprika, and onion powder. Put into a plastic bag. Coat potato wedges with oil and put into bag. Shake, and place onto a pizza pan. Bake 350° approximately 30 minutes or until tender.

RICE CASSEROLE

1/3 c. green pepper
1 medium onion
1 clove garlic
1 T. olive oil
2 c. chicken broth
1 T. Worcestershire sauce
1 c. long grain rice
3/4 t. salt

Heat oven to 350°. Sauté onion, pepper and garlic in oil. Add the rest of the ingredients and bake, covered for approximately 1 hour or until bubbly.

HASH BROWNS

1/2 c. chicken bouillon chicken broth
1 T. butter
3 potatoes

1 onion
1 green pepper
1 clove garlic
1/2 c. hot pepper (optional)

Shred potatoes and onion. Mince green pepper and garlic and add to the potatoes. Melt butter in a cast iron skillet. Add the vegetables, cover the pan and cook on low heat.
When potatoes begin sticking to the bottom of the skillet
add the chicken broth. Continue cooking on low heat until
potatoes are soft and cooked through.

BAKED GLAZED CARROTS

2 lbs. Carrots cut into 2-inch pieces
1 T. brown sugar
1/2 t. cinnamon
1/3 c. orange juice
1 T. melted butter
3/4 c. water

Heat oven to 350°. Place carrots in casserole dish.
Combine sugar, cinnamon, juice, butter and water. Pour
over carrots. Bake, uncovered, for 40 minutes. Cover and
bake another 15 minutes or until tender.

SCALLOPED CORN

1 bag frozen corn (fresh corn can be used)
22 saltine crackers (mashed)
1/2 c. milk
1/4 c. butter
1 t. sea salt
1/2 t. pepper

Mix above ingredients together and bake until bubbly, approximately 40 minutes. (If desired, sprinkle with paprika.)

COMPANY SCALLOPED CORN

1 package frozen corn
1/4 c. chopped pimento
1/4 c. chopped green pepper
1/8 c. chopped onion
1/2 c. milk
1/4 c. butter
14 saltine crackers (crushed)
1 t. sea salt
1/2 t. pepper

Combine above ingredients, reserving 1/2 c. crushed crackers. Sprinkle crackers over casserole. Bake 350° until bubbly, approximately 45 minutes.

SCALLOPED POTATOES

6 medium potatoes
3 T. butter
2 T. corn starch
2 1/2 c. skim milk
1/4 c. chopped onion
1/4 c. chopped green pepper (optional)
1 T. butter

Slice potatoes. Melt 3 T. butter in a saucepan, adding the flour, salt and pepper. Cook until bubbly. Slowly add the milk, heating until thickened, stirring constantly. Layer vegetables and sauce in casserole dish. Dot 1 T. butter over top of vegetables. Cover and bake 350°, approximately 40 minutes.

CREAMED ONIONS

2 pounds onions
1/4 c. fat free Parmesan cheese
1 T. butter
3 T. corn starch
1 c. skim milk
1 t. sea salt
1/2 t. pepper

Cook onions in water until done. Melt butter, in saucepan. Add 1/2 c. of milk. Stir cornstarch into remainder 1/2 c. of milk and add to melted butter. Add salt and pepper, heating milk and cornstarch mixture, stirring constantly until thickened. Drain onions and add creamed milk. Stir in cheese. Serve.

SPINACH CASSEROLE

2 packages frozen chopped spinach
2 1/2 T. chopped onion
2 eggs, beaten
1 c. fat free Parmesan cheese
8 oz. fat free sour cream
1 1/2 c. Spelt or vegetable spaghetti, cooked

Combine above ingredients in a casserole dish. Bake at 350° until bubbly.

Bibliography

Absorption and Utilization of Amino Acids, Mendel Friedman, ed. U.S. Department of Agriculture, Albany NY vol. I, II, III, CRC Press, Boca Raton, FL, 1989.

Acherio A, Rimm EB, Giovannucci EL, Spegelman D, Stampfer M, and Willett WC. "Dietary fat and risk of coronary heart disease in men." Brit Med J 313:84-90 (1996)

Alexander, J. W., B. B. MacMillan, J. D. Stinnett, C. K. Ogle, R. C. Bozian, J. E. Fischer, J. B. Oakes, M J. Morris, and R. Krummel "Beneficial Effects of Aggressive Protein Feeding in Severely Burned Children," Annals of Surgery 192: 505, 1980.

Allred JB. :too much of a good thing? An over-emphasis on eating lowfat food may be contributing to the alarming increase in overweight amount US adults." J Am Dietetic Assoc 95: 417-418 (1995)

Alpha-tocopherol Beta-carotene Cancer Prevention Study Group. "The effect of Vitamin E and Beta-carotene on the incidence of lung cancer and other cancers in male smokers." New Engl J Med 334: 1150-1155 (1996)

Balch, J. F. & Balch, P. A. Prescription for Nutritional Healing. New York: Avery Publishing Group, 1990.

Baldessarini, R. J. "Drugs and Treatment of Psychiatric Disorders," In: L. S. Goodman and A. Gilman, eds., The Pharmacologic Basis of Therapeutics, 7th ed., New York: MacMillan, 1985.

Boland, E. W. "Psychogenic Rheumatism: The Musculoskeletal Expression of Psychoneurosis," Annual of Rheumatological Disorders 6: 195, 1947.

Bucci, L. R. "Reversal of Osteoarthritis by Nutritional Intervention." ACA Journal of Chiropractic 27(November 1990): 69-72.

Buchwald, D., et al. "The Chronic, Active Epstein-Barr Virus Infection Syndrome and Primary Fibromyal-gia," Arthritis Rheumatology 30: 1132, 1987.

Campbell LV, Marmot PE, Dyer JA Borkman M, and Storlien LH. "The high-monounsaturated fat diet as a practical alternative for non-insulin dependent diabetes mellitus. " Diabetes Care 17:177-182 (1994)

Carper, J. Stop Aging Now. 1st ed. New York: Harper Collins Publishers, 1995.

Clement, C. D., ed. Anatomy of the Human Body. 30th ed. Philadelphia: Lea and Febiger, 1985.

Cousins, Norman. Anatomy of an Illness: As Perceived by the Patient. New York, NY: W. W. Norton & Co., 1979.

Cousins, Norman. The Healing Heart. New York, NY: W.W. Norton & Co., 1983.

Crawford MA, Cunnane SC, and Harbige LS. "A new theory of evolution." In Essential Fatty Acids and Eicosanoids. Sinclair A and Gibson R eds. American Oil Chemists' Society Press. Champaign, IL (1993)

Daviglus ML, Stamler J, Orencia AJ Dyer AR, Liu K, Greenland P, walsh MK, Morris D, and shekelle RB. "Fish consumption and the 30-year risk of fatal myocardial infarction." N Engl J Med 336:1046-1053 (1997)

Dexter, P. and Brandt, K. "Distribution and Predictors of Depressive Symptoms of Osteoarthritis." Journal of Rheumatology 21(2): 279-286, 1994.

Elrod, J. M. The Body Advantage: Total Wellness System. Montgomery, AL: Dr. Joe M. Elrod and Associates, 1996.

Elrod, J. M. "How Not To Be a Dropout," Newsletter, Sportrooms of America, Vol. 3: 27, 1982.

Elrod, J.M. Reversing Fibromyalgia. Pleasant Grove, Ut.: Woodland Publishing, 1997.

Ferraccioli, G. F. et al. "EMG Biofeedback in Fibromyalgia Syndrome," Journal of Rheumatology 16: 1013, 1989.

Flatt JP. "Use and storage of carbohydrate and fat." Am J

Clin Nutr 61:952S-959S (1995)

Franceschi s, Favero A, Decarli D, Negri E, La Vecchia C, Fetratoni M, Russo A Salvini S, Amadori D, Conti E, Montella M, and Giacosa A. "Intake of Macronutrients and risk of breast cancer." Lancer 347:1351-1356 (1996)

Garg A, Grundy SM, and Koffler M. "Effect of high carbohydrate intake on hyperglycemia, islet function, and plasma lipoproteins in NIDDM. " Diabetes Care 15:1572-1580 (1992)

Garnett, L. R. "Strong Medicine," Harvard Health Letter, pp. 4-6, 1995.

Goldenberg, D. L. "Fibromyalgia and Chronic Fatigue Syndrome: Are They the Same?" Journal of Musculoskeletal Medicine 7: 19, 1990.

Goldenberg, D. L. et al. "The Impact of Cognitive-Behavioral Therapy on Fibromyalgia," Arthritis Rheumatology 34(suppl 9): S190, 1991.

Golay KL, Allaz AF, Morel Y de Tonnac N, Tankova S, and Reaven G. " Similar weight loss with low- or high-carbohydrate diets." Am J Clin Nutr 63:174-178 (1996)

Hauri, P. and D. R. Hawkins "Alpha-Delta Sleep," Electroenceph Clin Neurophysiology 34:233, 1973.

Hendler, N. and Kolodny, A. L. "Using Medication Wisely in Chronic Pain," Patient Care, 6:125-139, May, 1992.

Hendler, S. S., M.D. The Doctor's Vitamin and Mineral Encyclopedia. New York: Simon and Schuster, 1990.

Hess, E. V., M.D. and A. Mòngey, M.D. "Drug-Related Lupus," Bulletin on the Rheumatic Diseases 40(August 1991): 1-7.

Lands WEM. Fish and human health. Academic Press. Orlando, FL. (1986)

Lanting CI, Fidler V, Huisman M, Touwen BCL, and Boersma ER. "Neurological differences between 9-year-old children fed breastmilk or formula-milk as babies. " Lancet 344:1319-1322 (1994)

McGee H. On Food and Cooking. MacMillan Publishing. New York. (1984)

Mohr A, Bowry VW, and Srocker R. "Dietary supplementation with coenzyme Q10 results in increased levels of ubiquninol-10 within circulating lipoproteins to the initiation of lipid peroxidation." Biochem Biphys Acta 1126:247-254 (1992)

Moldofsky, H. D. et al. "Musculoskeletal Symptoms and Non-REM Sleep Disturbance in Patients with 'Fibrositis Syndrome' and Healthy Subjects," Psychosomatic Medicine 37:341, 1975.

Moldofsky, H. D. "Sleep, Neuroimmune and Neuroendocrine Functions in Fibromyalgia and Chronic Fatigue Syndrome," Advances in Neuroimmunology 5:39-56, 1995.

Omenn GS, Goodman Ge, Thornquist MD, Balmes J, Cullen MR, Glass A, Keogh JP, Meyskens, FL, Valanis R, Williams JH, Barnhart S, and Hammar S. "Effects of a combination of betacarotene and vitamin A on lung cancer and cardiovascular disease. " New Engl J Med 334:1150-1155 (1996)

Parillo M, Rivellese AA, Ciardullo AZ, Capaldo B, Giacco A, Genovese S, and Riccardi G. "A high-monounsaturated fat/low-carbohydrate diet improves peripheral insulin sensitivity in non-insulin-dependent diabetic patients." Metabol 41:1373-1378 (1993)

Quillin, P. "The Role of Nutrition in Cancer Treatment," Health Councilor 4(6).

Quillin, P. Healing Nutrients, Contemporary Books, Inc., Chicago, IL, 1987.

Rimm EB, Stampger MJ, Ascherio A, Giovannucci E, Colditz GA, and Willett WC. " Vitamin E consumption and risk of coronary heart disease in men." New Engl J Med 328: 1450-1456 (1993)

Roberts HJ. Aspartame. Is it Safe ? Charles Press.

Philadelphia, PA (1990)

Simms, R. W. et al. "Lack of Association Between Fibromyalgia Syndrome and Abnormalities in Muscle Energy Metabolism," Arthritis Rheumatology 37:801-807, 1994.

Weil, A., M.D. Natural Health, Natural Medicine. Boston: Houghton Mifflin, 1990.

Weintraub, S., N.D. Natural Treatments for ADD and Hyperactivity. Pleasant Grove, UT: Woodland Publishing, 1997.

Wolever TMS, Jenkins DJA, Jenkins AL, and Josse RG. "The glycemic index: methodology and clinical implications. " Am J Clin Nutr 54:846-854 (1991)

Resource List

The Fibromyalgia Network
P.O. Box 31750
Tucson, AZ 85751-1750
800-853-2929 or FAX 520-290-5550.

The American Fibromyalgia Syndrome Association, Inc.
6380 E Tanque Verde Rd. Ste. D,
Tucson, AZ 85715
520-733-1570

Fibromyalgia Association of Central Ohio
P.O. Box 21988
Columbus OH 43221-0988
614-457-4222

American Association for Chronic Fatigue Syndrome
7 Van Buren Street
Albany, NY 12206
518-482-2202

Fibromyalgia Association of Greater Washington, Inc.
12210 Fairfax Towne Center, Ste. 500
Fairfax, VA 22033
703-790-2324

Fibromyalgia Association of Texas
3810 Keele Dr.
Garland, TX 75041
214-271-5085

Inland Northwest Fibromyalgia Assoc.
9209 E. Mission, Ste. B
Spokane, WA 99206
509-921-7741

Fibromyalgia Times
P.O. Box 20408
Columbus, OH 43221-0990
614-457-4222

Fibromyalgia Frontiers
P.O. Box 2373
Centreville, OH 22020
703-912-1727

Arthritis Foundation
P.O. Box 19000
Atlanta, GA 30326
800-283-7800

Fibromyalgia Educational Systems
500 Bushaway Road
Wayzata, MN 55391
612-473-6218 or 419-843-3153

The CFIDS Association of America, Inc.
P.O. Box 220398
Charlotte, NC 28222-0398
800-442-3437

Massachusetts CFIDS Association
808 Main Street
Waltham, MA 02154
617-893-4415

Restless Legs Syndrome Foundation, Inc.
304 Glenwood Ave.
Raleigh, NC 27603-1455
919-834-0821

Seattle Fibromyalgia International Team, Inc.
P.O. Box 77373
Seattle, WA 98177
206-362-2310

The TMJ Association
6418 W. Washington Blvd.
Milwaukee, WI 53213
414-259-3223

Fibromyalgia Association of BC
Box 15455
Vancouver, BC V6B 5B2 Canada
604-430-6643

The Ontario Fibromyalgia Association
250 Bloor Street, E. Ste. 901
Toronto, ON V4W 3P2 Canada

The Arthritis Society, BC Division
805 West 10th Avenue
Vancouver, BC V5Z 1L7 Canada
604-879-7511

American Association for Marriage and Family Therapy
1133 15th St. NW, Ste. 300
Washington, DC 20005
800-374-2638

American Psychiatric Association, APA
Department AT, 1400 K St. NW
Washington DC 20005
202-682-6220

GSWG, Getting Well Support Groups
6101 Nall Avenue
Mission, Kansas 66202
913-432-HOPE (4673) fax: 913-384-2464

Depression, Awareness, Recognition and Treatment
(D/ART)
5600 Fishcers Lane, Rm. 10-85
Rockville, MD 20857
800-421-4211

National Alliance for the Mentally Ill
200 N. Bleve Rd., Ste. 1015
Arlington, VA 22203-3754
800-950-6264

National Association of Social Workers
750 First St. NE, Ste. 700
Washington, DC 20002
202-408-8600

National Depressive and Manic Depressive Association
730 N. Franklin, Ste. 501
Chicago, IL 60610
800-82N-DMDA or 800-826-3632

National Foundation for Depressive Illlness
P.O. Box 2257
New York, NY 10116
800-248-4344

National Mental Health Association
1021 Prince St.
Alexandria, VA 22314-2971
800-969-6642

American Academy of Allergy and Immunology
611 E. Wells St.
Milwaukee, WI 53202
414-272-6071

American Academy of Environmental Medicine
P.O. Box 16105
Denver, CO 80216
303-622-9755

American Apitherapy Society
P.O. Box 74
North Hartland, VT 05052
802-295-8764

American Association of Acupuncture and Oriental
Medicine
4101 Lake Boone Tr., Ste. 201
Raleigh, NC 27607
919-787-5181

American College of Rheumatology
60 Executive Park S., Ste. 150
Atlanta, GA 30329
404-633-3777

American Dietetic Association
430 N. Michigan Ave.
Chicago, IL 60611

American Holistic Medical Association
2002 Eastlake Ave. E.
Seattle, WA 98102
206-322-6842
American Nutritionists Association
P.O. Box 34030
Bethesda, MD 20817

Ankylosing Spondylitis Association
511 N. LaCienega Blvd., Ste. 216
Los Angeles, CA 90048
800-777-8189
310-652-0609 (in California)

Arthritis Foundation
1314 Spring St. NW
Atlanta, GA 30309
800-283-7800

Food Allergy Network
4744 Holly Ave.
Fairfax, VA 22030-5647
703-691-3179

Lupus Foundation of America
4 Research Pl., Ste. 180
Rockville, MD 20850-3226
800-558-0121

National Chronic Pain Outreach Association
7979 Old Georgetown Rd., Ste. 100
Bethesda, MD 20814
301-652-4948

National Commission for the Certification of
Acupuncturists
1424 16th St. NW, Ste. 501
Washington, DC 20036
202-232-1404

National Institute of Arthritis and Musculoskeletal and
Skin Diseases
NIH Information Clearinghouse
Box AMS
8000 Rockville Pike
Bethesda, MD 20892
301-495-4484

National Institute of Arthritis and Musculoskeletal and
Skin Diseases Multipurpose Centers

Middle Atlantic

Cornell University Medical College
The Hospital for Special Surgery
Research Building, Room 605
535 East 70th St.
New York, NY 10021
212-606-1189

Midwest

Case Western Reserve University
2074 Abington Rd.
Cleveland, OH 44106
216-844-3168

Indiana University School of Medicine
541 Clinical Dr., Room 492
Indianapolis, IN 46202-5103
317-274-4225

Northwestern University Medical School
303 E. Chicago Ave., Ward 3-315
Chicago, IL 60611
313-503-8197

New England

Brigham and Women's Hospital
75 Francis St.
Boston, MA 02115
617-732-5356

Boston University School of Medicine
71 E. Concord St., K5
Boston, MA 02118
617-638-4310

University of Connecticut School of Medicine
263 Farmington Ave.
Farmington, CT 06030-1310
203-679-3605

Pacific

Stanford University
100 Welch Rd., Ste. 203
Pal Alto, CA 94304

University of California, San Diego
Department of Medicine, 0945
La Jolla, CA 92093
619-558-1291

University of California, San Francisco
P.O. Box 0868
San Francisco, CA 94143-0868
415-750-2104

University of California School of Medicine
10833 LeConte Ave., 47-139 CHS
Los Angeles, CA 90024-1736
213-825-7991
South

University of Alabama at Birmingham
UAB Station, THT 429A
Birmingham, AL 35294
205-934-5306

University of North Carolina at Chapel Hill
932 FLOB, UNC-CH School of Medicine
Chapel Hill, NC 27514
919-966-4191

Other Resource Materials

The Body Advantage (1996), by Dr. Joe M. Elrod: Elastic stretch exercise device including video with complete exercise program designed specifically for fibromyalgia and arthritic sufferers. To order: Call (334) 272-3605, fax (334) 279-3117, send email to drjoeelrod@reversingfibromyalgia.com, or write to 3066 Zelda Road, Suite 212, Montgomery, AL 36106.

The Success Journal, Elrod, Dr. Joe M. Kinner Printing/Dr. Joe M. Elrod & Associates, 1996. To order: Call (334) 272-3605 or write to 3066 Zelda Road, Suite 212, Montgomery, AL 36106.

To contact Dr. Elrod regarding consultation, speaking engagements, or for other information, use the following:

Dr. Joe M. Elrod
3066 Zelda Rd. Suite 212
Montgomery, Alabama 36106
phone: (334) 272-3605
fax: (334) 279-3117
email: drjoeelrod@worldnet.att.net
website: http://www.reversingfibromyalgia.com

Fibromyalgia Cookbook, A Daily Guide to Become Healthy Again: A four-month, daily guide to making lifestyle changes which help the immune system as it heals. Includes information on nutritional changes, an exercise program, acupressure points, herbs and other helpful ideas on natural ways to help with symptoms as the body heals.

To order: Call Fibromyalgia Solutions, 816-628-5427 or write to: Fibromyalgia Solutions, 305 E 9th Street, Kearney, MO 64060. Cost $15.00 plus $3.00 for shipping and handling. Visit our website: www.kcnet.com/fms

"Fibromyalgia, Conquering the Challenge": Audio tape set containing much of the information presented in the of half-day seminars sponsored by Fibromyalgia Solutions. Includes information about fibromyalgia, what triggers symptoms, information on rebuilding the immune system, natural ways to help with pain, ways to get a better night sleep, and much much more. To order: Fibromyalgia Solutions, 305 E 9th Street, Kearney, MO 64060. 816-628-5427. Cost $16.00 (Set of two tapes) plus $3.00 for shipping and handling. Visit our website: www.kcnet.com/fms

"Conquering the Challenge Fibromyalgia Newsletter": This bi-monthly newsletter features a variety of information from support issues to the latest in research. To order: Call 913-432-HOPE (913-432-4673) or write GWSG 6101 Nall Avenue, Mission, Kansas, 66202. Cost $16.00/yr. (6 issues).